Radiology
for
MRCP

Cases with discussion

Radiology
for
MRCP

Cases with discussion

Second edition

Sarah J Howling
MBBS MRCP FRCR
Consultant Radiologist and
Honorary Senior Lecturer
The Whittington Hospital
Highgate Hill
London N19 5NF

Alan Grundy
MB ChB DCH FRCR
Consultant and Senior Lecturer
in Diagnostic Radiology
St George's Hospital and
Medical School
London

Paul J Jenkins
MA BChir MRCP
Reader in Endocrinology
Consultant Physician
St Bartholomew's and the
Royal London Hospital

Rema Kaur Wasan
MA MBBS MRCP FRCR
Consultant Radiologist
King's College Hospital
London

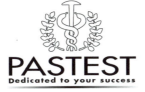

PASTEST
Dedicated to your success

© 2003 PasTest Ltd
Egerton Court
Parkgate Estate
Knutsford
Cheshire WA16 8DX

Telephone: 01565 752000

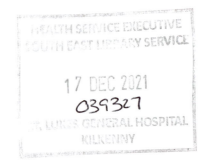
First published 1998
Reprinted 1999
Second edition 2003

ISBN: 1 901198 22 7

A catalogue record for this book is available from the British Library.

The information contained within this book was obtained by the authors from reliable sources. However, while every effort has been made to ensure its accuracy, no responsibility for loss, damage or injury occasioned to any person acting or refraining from action as a result of information contained herein can be accepted by the publisher or the authors.

PasTest Revision Books and Intensive Courses
PasTest has been established in the field of postgraduate medical education since 1972, providing revision books and intensive study courses for doctors preparing for their professional examinations. Books and courses are available for the following specialties:

MRCGP, MRCP Part 1 and Part 2, MRCPCH Part 1 and Part 2, MRCOG, DRCOG, MRCS, MRCPsych, DCH, FRCA and PLAB.

For further details contact:

PasTest Ltd, Freepost, Knutsford, Cheshire, WA16 7BR
Tel: 01565 752000   Fax: 01565 650264
Email: enquiries@pastest.co.uk
Web site: www.pastest.co.uk

Cover design by Elaine Moore
Text prepared by Vision Typesetting, Manchester
Printed and bound in Great Britain by Page Bros (Norwich) Ltd

Contents

Foreword

Over the last two decades Radiology, as an imaging science, has witnessed enormous advances, particularly in the field of axial imaging and interventional techniques. The specialty has moved from one of static imaging of normal/morbid anatomy, portraying macroscopic pathology with the aid of X-rays, to more dynamic techniques which may offer insight into the pathophysiology of disease. From the basement reporting room of old to the modern radiology conference room, multidisciplinary meetings are now a forum for the meeting of our clinical colleagues in medicine and surgery together with histologists, oncologists and radiotherapists to discuss and decide on best patient management.

Reflecting these advances, standard textbooks of radiology are a formidable size and so, for MRCP preparation, impractical in terms of obtaining a good basic balanced knowledge of radiology. It was clearly with this in mind that the first edition of *Radiology for MRCP* was conceived and, very successfully was able to encompass, through the cases and discussions of differential diagnosis, huge tracts of radiology most likely to be encountered in the MRCP examination.

The second edition, with Drs Grundy and Wasan joining the original authors Drs Howling and Jenkins, has expanded the number of cases. There is a change of format with each case having an 'MCQ style' question with possible answers and, as previously, followed by discussion of the answer together with critical evaluation of differential diagnoses and related conditions.

All four authors are well known as committed and dedicated teachers. In the essential first section they guide the readers through the normal anatomy of the different imaging modalities and the importance of following a routine in the interpretation of films. The 126 cases all have an exceptional reproduction of the original radiographs – many with supplementary images. The style and 'easy readability' of the text makes for compulsive reading so that, once started, it is difficult to put the book down. There is clearly an emphasis on plain films for analysis – reflecting their continuing importance in diagnosis – but with a careful balance of other imaging modalities with an excellent commentary on technical aspects as for CT and MRI.

In addition to enabling the readers to 'graft' an excellent working radiological knowledge, in the form of images, to their MRCP reading, the text also serves as part revision for the conditions discussed.

The authors are to be commended on this book which is a **must** in terms of the required radiological information for MRCP preparation.

Huw Walters FRCR
Clinical Director of Radiology
King's College Hospital
London

Preface

Candidates now preparing for the MRCP Part 2 examination need to be familiar with an ever-increasing array of imaging techniques. Although 'conventional' imaging remains the mainstay of most diagnostic imaging, there has been an increase in the use of computed tomography (CT)and magnetic resonance imaging (MRI)and this has been reflected in the types and proportions of cases encountered in the written exam.

When teaching MRCP candidates, it has become clear that access to the fundamentals of these newer imaging modalities is limited, without reference to hefty radiological texts. The cases in this book, together with many supplementary radiographs, use all the relevant imaging modalities and encompass the majority of examination questions that the candidate is likely to face in both the slide section and grey cases. In most cases there is a specific answer, but in some a differential diagnosis is required. All questions are followed by a discussion and details of similar conditions that the candidate should be familiar with. This additional information may be ignored as the exam approaches, as all answers are readily identified by bold type.

Success in the examination depends on exposure to a large number of cases, which both familiarises the candidate with the radiology of more common diseases and also encourages a stratagem for approaching those cases that are not immediately familiar. Such a stratagem is essential if all the abnormalities are to be identified on each film. It is certainly easier to see an abnormality if one is looking for it, e.g. the finding of multiple pulmonary nodules should prompt a search for rib destruction, mastectomy and mediastinal lymph adenopathy which might not otherwise be immediately apparent.

It is recommended that the candidate first reads the section on the interpretation of images at the front of this book, which is devoted to helping the reader understand the principles of interpretation, both of plain films and other imaging modalities. When appropriate, the candidate is referred to more detailed radiological texts for additional information.

Acknowledgements

The authors would like to thank Dr Katherine Miszkiel of the National Hospital for Nervous Diseases and Neurosurgery, Queens Square, London, Dr Chris Hare of the Middlesex Hospital, London and Dr Hugh Sansom of the Chelsea and Westminster Hospital, London who so willingly provided some of the radiographs reproduced here. We also thank the Department of Medical Photography at St Bartholomew's Hospital, London and St George's Hospital, London who prepared the photographic prints.

Sarah Howling   **Alan Grundy**
Paul Jenkins   **Rema Wasan**

Guidance on how to interpret the different types of imaging modalities

There is no single fixed method by which to evaluate the different types of imaging currently available. What matters is to follow a routine. What follows is the authors' own suggested scheme, with a few helpful tips on reviewing the central imaging modalities. Candidates can modify these sequences for themselves.

The chest radiograph

This remains one of the most difficult plain films to interpret, and an ordered approach is essential (Figure i).

1. Technical factors: if the film is well centred, the medial ends of the clavicles are equidistant from the vertebral spinous processes. Observe the side marker and if dextrocardia is present look closely for possible bronchiectasis.

2. Trachea: if the trachea is not central it may be deviated away from a superior mediastinal mass (in most cases a retrosternal goitre) or pulled over to the side of the lesion by fibrosis or a decreased lung volume. The normal carinal angle (60–75°) may be widened by an enlarged left atrium or enlarged subcarinal lymph nodes. On the right the tracheal margin can be traced down to the right main bronchus. This border is known as the right paratracheal stripe (normally no more than 5 mm wide). Widening may be due to mediastinal tumours, pleural effusions, lymphadenopathy or mediastinitis.

3. Heart and mediastinum: the position of the heart is variable. On average, one third lies to the right of the midline. The usual cardiothoracic ratio, i.e. the ratio of the transverse cardiac diameter to the internal transverse thoracic diameter is less than 1:2. An increase in the transverse cardiac diameter of

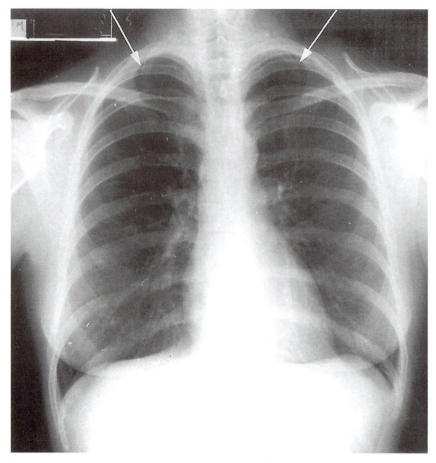

Figure i: Normal chest radiograph. Note incidental bilateral cervical ribs (arrows).

1.5 cm between successive radiographs is significant. Note that apparent cardiac enlargement occurs on expiration, in the supine and AP projections and when the diaphragms are elevated. All borders of the heart and mediastinum should be clearly defined, except where the heart sits on the left hemidiaphragm. A search should be made for fluid levels, abnormal densities, mediastinal emphysema and calcifications.

4. Hilar regions: they should be of equal density and size with concave lateral borders. Normally the left hilum is 0.5–2 cm higher than the right. Only the pulmonary arteries and upper lobe veins contribute significantly to the hilar shadows on a chest radiograph.

5. Lungs: the only structures that can be visualised within normal lungs are the blood vessels, interlobar fissures and the walls of certain larger bronchi seen end on. By comparing one lung with the other, zone by zone, areas of abnormality are easier to detect. A useful rule on the lateral view is that there should be an increase in relative transradiancy as the eye travels down the thoracic vertebral bodies.

6. **Fissures:** on the PA view, only the horizontal fissure is seen. It runs from the right hilum to the region of the sixth rib in the axillary line.

7. **Diaphragm:** in most patients the right hemidiaphragm is higher than the left. On full inspiration the normal right hemidiaphragm is at the level of the sixth rib anteriorly. Loss of outline indicates that adjacent tissue has become non-air containing, e.g. lower lobe consolidation. Only the superior surface is seen unless a pneumoperitoneum is present.

8. **Soft tissues:** in females check that both breasts are present.

9. **Bones:** a survey should be made of all the bones. In particular, check the ribs for notching or destruction.

10. **Below the diaphragm:** a search should be made for free intraperitoneal gas, abscesses, dilated bowel loops and a displaced gastric bubble. Calcified hepatic tumours, granulomas and gallstones may be seen.

11. **Hidden areas:** special attention should be paid to the lung apices and behind the heart.

Useful tips

- The silhouette sign permits localisation of a lesion on a PA film. An intrathoracic opacity, if in contact with a border of the heart, mediastinum or diaphragm will obscure that border, e.g. lesions of the right middle lobe or lingula will obscure the right and left cardiac borders, respectively. If, on the other hand, a border is retained and the abnormality is superimposed then it must be either anterior or posterior.
- A well-defined mass seen above the clavicles is always posterior.
- An air bronchogram indicates that shadowing is intrapulmonary.

The abdominal radiograph

1. **Gas pattern and position:** relatively large amounts of gas are usually present in the stomach and colon of a normal patient, with relatively small amounts in the small bowel which are rarely sufficient to outline the whole of a loop. Short fluid levels in the small and large bowel are a normal finding. The calibre of the colon is extremely variable. However, in inflammatory bowel disease a transverse colonic diameter of 5.5 cm is taken as the upper limit of normal. Look for any abnormal positioning of bowel loops which may (for example) indicate the presence of an abdominal mass.

2. **Gas outside the bowel lumen:** including inspection of the biliary tree, portal venous system, bowel wall and genitourinary system.

3. Ascites: should be looked for in addition to any abnormal opacities. Large masses arising from the pelvis may be due to an enlarged bladder or may be ovarian or uterine in origin.

4. Abdominal viscera: identify the lower borders of the liver and spleen, renal outlines and psoas muscles. Note the presence of any calcification and attempt to localise.

5. Bones: not forgetting the vertebral bodies, sacroiliac joints and femoral heads.

Useful tips:

- Visualisation of the inner as well as the outer bowel wall – 'Rigler's sign', is a valuable indication of a pneumoperitoneum.
- Dilatation of the bowel occurs in mechanical obstruction, paralytic ileus, acute ischaemia and inflammatory bowel disease.
- The most common abdominal calcifications are of little clinical significance and include phleboliths, calcified lymph nodes, costal cartilages and arterial calcification.
- Substantial enlargement of the liver has to occur before it can be detected on a plain radiograph.

The hand X-ray

Observe:

1. Bone density: whether normal, increased or decreased, and if abnormal, whether focal or diffuse.

2. Soft tissues: look for swellings, loss of soft tissues and calcifications.

3. Joints: assess the joint space and look specifically for erosions. If erosions are present note their site in relation to individual joints, distribution and whether symmetrical.

4. Terminal tufts: inspect for erosions.

5. Alignment and deformities, e.g. short metacarpals, ulnar deviation.

6. Look specifically for chondrocalcinosis, particularly in the region of the triangular fibrocartilage of the wrist joint.

The skull X-ray

The bones of the normal skull vault have an inner and outer table of compact bone with spongy bone (diploë) between them. The sutures remain visible even when fused and blood vessels cause impressions on the bones of the vault.

1. **Look for intracranial calcifications,** most of which are normal and of no clinical significance. The position of the calcified pineal gland (seen on approximately two-thirds of adult skull films) is the only means of identifying the midline. A deviation of more than 3 mm from the midline on the frontal view is abnormal.

2. **Review the bones** of the vault and skull base for areas of lysis or sclerosis.

3. **Examine the pituitary fossa.** Normal dimensions are: depth 8–12 mm; widest AP diameter 11–16 mm. Enlargement or ballooning is most commonly due to tumours of the pituitary. The dorsum sella may be eroded in prolonged raised intracranial pressure.

4. **Inspect the paranasal air sinuses.**

Intravenous urogram (IVU)

1. **Plain film:** identify all calcifications which will be obscured by contrast. The major causes of urinary tract calcification are: urinary calculi, nephrocalcinosis, localised calcification due to conditions such as tuberculosis or tumours and prostatic calcification (Figure ii).

2. **Position of the kidneys:** the left kidney is generally higher than the right. Their axes should be parallel to the outer margins of the psoas muscles. If abnormal, the cause is most often congenital malposition or displacement by a retroperitoneal mass.

3. **Renal size:** renal length generally approximates to 3–3.5 lumbar vertebrae plus their discs. The left kidney is often slightly larger than the right but a discrepancy of more than 1.5 cm between the two sides is suspicious.

4. **Renal shape and outline:** if any indentations or bulges are present they must be explained. The renal parenchymal width should be uniform and symmetrical. A bulge of the renal outline usually indicates a mass and is generally associated with displacement and deformity of the adjacent calices. (An important normal variant causing a bulge of the left renal outline is the so-called 'splenic hump'.)

5. **The calices:** they should be reasonably symmetrical and evenly distributed. A normal calix is cup-shaped. A dilated calix is referred to as 'clubbed'. Caliceal dilatation has two basic causes: (i) obstruction – dilatation of the collecting system down to the obstructing lesion and (ii) destruction of the papilla, which may be due to chronic pyelonephritis, tuberculosis, papillary necrosis or obstructive atrophy.

6. **Renal pelves:** look for filling defects, the causes of which include calculi, blood clot, tumours and sloughed papillae.

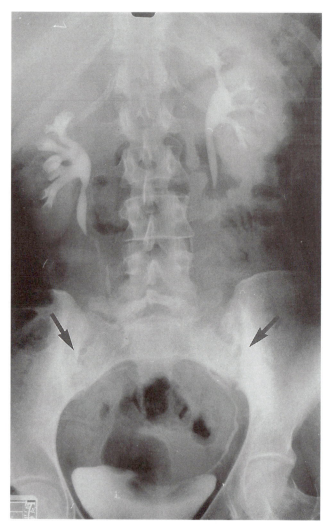

Figure ii: Normal IVU. The smooth indentation on the bladder is due to the normal uterus. Note bilateral sacroiliitis (arrows) in this patient with a history of inflammatory bowel disease.

7. **Ureters:** Only part of their length is usually seen on any one film. Dilatation is usually due to obstruction. Look also for displacement.

8. **The bladder:** shape, size and outline, which should be smooth. After micturition the bladder should be empty.

Barium examinations

1. To distinguish between a small-bowel follow-through, in which serial films are taken after the ingestion of barium, and a small-bowel enema, in which barium is injected through a nasojejunal tube, look for the presence of a tube which indicates that the latter has been performed. Small bowel: check the bowel calibre. A diameter of greater than 30 mm is definitely abnormal. Dilatation of small bowel usually indicates malabsorption, paralytic ileus or small-bowel obstruction. Look for strictures, which must be differentiated from normal peristalsis. A smooth tapering stricture is more likely to be benign, whereas one ending abruptly, with overhanging edges giving an appearance termed 'shouldering' is more likely to be malignant. This rule is also pertinent to large-bowel studies. Inspect the mucosal folds, checking both their thickness (normally no more than 2 mm) and frequency (generally 1–6 mm apart). Small bowel folds become thickened in numerous conditions, including malabsorption, infiltration, inflammatory bowel disease and oedema of the bowel wall. Filling defects may be intraluminal, e.g. *Ascaris lumbricoides*; arise from the bowel wall, e.g. carcinoma; or extraluminal, causing wall compression, e.g. pancreatic mass.

2. Look for alteration in position of bowel loops.

3. Large bowel: note that haustra can normally be recognised in the whole of the colon but may be absent in the descending and sigmoid regions. Strictures in the large bowel are generally due to diverticular disease, Crohn's disease or ischaemic colitis and less commonly tuberculosis, radiation or lymphoma.

4. Do not forget to look outside the bowel for additional diagnostic clues, e.g. sacroiliitis, gallstones or a bamboo spine.

Computed tomography

Lesions of high attenuation on CT are white and have high CT values (Hounsfield Units/HU). High attenuation areas on unenhanced scans are typically due to haemorrhage (+55 to +75 HU) or calcification (+400 to +1000 HU).

Conversely, low attenuation lesions are black and have low or negative CT values. Tissues with low Hounsfield Units include air (–1000 HU), fat (–100 to –60 HU) and to a lesser degree water (0 HU).

Determining the Hounsfield Units for an undiagnosed lesion gives useful information on its composition.

• **Abdomen**

Normal appearances are demonstrated in Figure iii. A useful approach may be

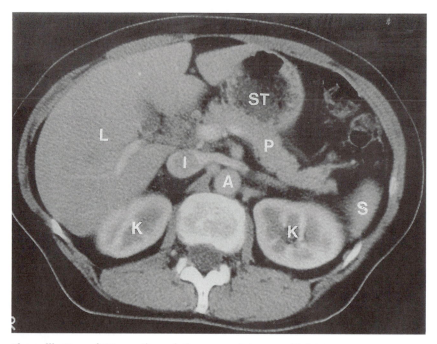

Figure iii: Normal CT scan through the upper abdomen with intravenous contrast. Liver (L), Kidneys (K), Tip of spleen (S), Pancreas (P), Stomach (ST), Aorta (A) and Inferior vena cava (I).

to evaluate each viscus in turn, after noting whether intravenous contrast has been given (usually indicated by the abbreviation '+C') by quickly inspecting the aorta and inferior vena cava. Familiarise yourself with the normal pre- and post-contrast appearances and the density of fluid on CT (see Case 112).

Points to remember include:

1. Liver: the normal hepatic parenchyma prior to contrast enhancement has a higher density than muscle and is higher or equal in density to the spleen. The hepatic veins are seen as low density branching structures. This difference in density between the liver and spleen is accentuated by haemochromatosis and reversed by fatty infiltration. Normal intrahepatic bile ducts are not visible. Intravenous contrast is often given to emphasise the density difference between normal parenchyma and lesions which enhance poorly, e.g. most abscesses, metastases or haematomas.

2. Spleen: many conditions which result in enlargement of the spleen cause no change in its density on CT, e.g. portal hypertension.

3. Renal tract: basic principles of interpretation are the same as with the IVU. The ureters are seen as small dots in cross-section lying on the psoas muscles.

CT is useful to assess renal masses, trauma, infarction and neoplastic infiltration.

4. Adrenal glands: the right adrenal gland lies immediately behind the inferior vena cava, whereas the left adrenal gland is normally medial to the upper pole of the left kidney. A limb thickness greater than a diaphragmatic crus (or >10 mm) is suspicious. The adrenal glands comprise a 'body' and two 'limbs', which form an inverted V or Y shape.

In addition to inspecting the viscera, check for ascites (fluid density surrounding the viscera), lymphadenopathy (particularly in the region of the major blood vessels), aortic aneurysm and do not forget the vertebral bodies and paraspinal regions where a psoas abscess may be lurking.

- **Brain**

1. Ascertain whether contrast has been given. It tends not to be given in patients with suspected head injury or who are suspected of recent cerebral haemorrhage.

2. Check for symmetry of the lateral ventricles and midline structures.

3. Check ventricular size. Two basic mechanisms may cause the ventricles to enlarge: (i) obstruction to the flow of cerebrospinal fluid (CSF) and (ii) secondary to atrophy of brain tissue.

4. Compare any abnormal tissue density with the normal surrounding brain. High attenuation (white) is seen with recent haemorrhage, calcification and areas of contrast enhancement. Low attenuation (black) is usually due to neoplasms or infarcts or is due to oedema which commonly surrounds tumours, infarcts, haematomas and areas of inflammation. Oedema does not enhance with intravenous contrast.

5. Do not forget to inspect the sinuses and orbits.

As a rule it is not possible to diagnose the nature of a mass on the basis of attenuation values alone (an exception being lipoma).

MRI basics

- Axial, coronal and sagittal projections are all possible. Since no signal is produced from bone, there is no bone artefact and hence MRI is superior to CT in examination of the posterior fossa and spinal cord structures.
- Different sequences change the signal intensities of visualised structures. On T1-weighted images (Figure iv), CSF appears **black** and fat appears **white**. On T2-weighted images (Figure v), CSF appears **white**.
- High signal refers to structures that are white and, conversely, low signal structures are black.

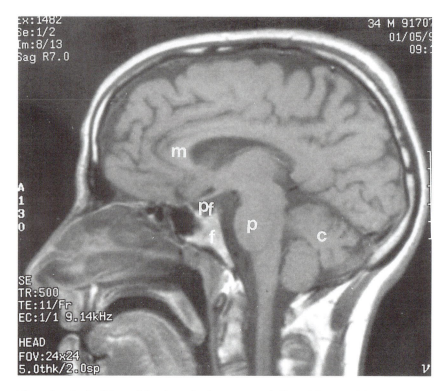

Figure iv: Sagittal T1-weighted MRI brain scan. Cerebellum (C), Pons (P), Corpus callosum (M), Pituitary fossa (PF), Fat in marrow of clivus (F).

- The natural differences in signal intensity are sufficiently great that contrast is needed much less often with MRI than with CT. If gadolinium DTPA (contrast medium) is given then a T1-weighted sequence is performed and enhancing tissues show up as white or high signal. Enhancement implies breakdown of the blood–brain barrier.
- MRI does not show calcification or bone detail for which CT is superior.
- Principles of diagnosis are similar to CT, in that the basic signs to look for are a change in signal intensity and evidence of mass effect.

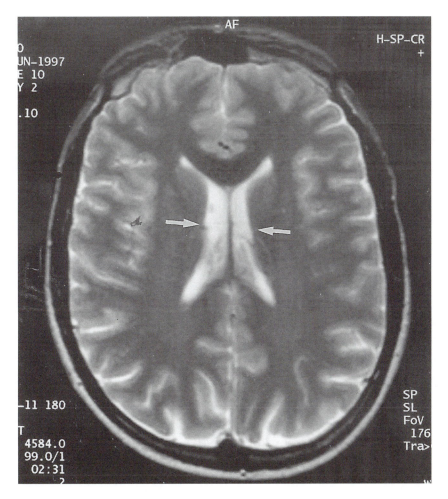

Figure v: Axial T2-weighted MRI brain scan at the level of the bodies of the lateral ventricles (arrows).

Bibliography

Grainger and Allison's Diagnostic Radiology: A Textbook of Medical Imaging.
Grainger et al., Churchill Livingstone 4th ed., 2001
All aspects of radiology are covered. A useful reference text.

Clinical Imaging. An Atlas of Differential Diagnosis. Eisenberg RL (1996) 3rd
ed., Lippincott–Raven
A well structured text which provides a differential radiological diagnosis
for all the conditions and signs that the candidate is likely to encounter. All
imaging modalities are covered and there are multiple useful illustrations.

Bone and Joint Imaging. Resnick D (July 1996) WB Saunders
A reference guide for all aspects of bone and joint imaging.

Aids to Radiological Differential Diagnosis. Chapman S and Nakielny R
(1995) 3rd ed., WB Saunders
An excellent pocket reference book containing multiple, well explained and
useful lists but no radiographic illustrations.

Imaging of diseases of the chest. Armstrong P et al. (2000), Mosby.

Cases with questions, answers and discussion

Case 1

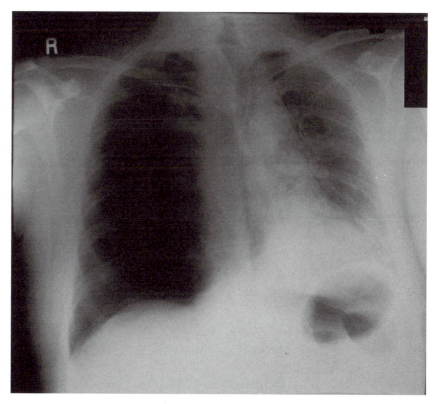

This 62-year-old man is acutely short of breath following laser therapy to an oesophageal carcinoma.

Question

1   What is the most likely diagnosis?
   ☐   A   Intraperitoneal perforation
   ☐   B   Left lower lobe collapse
   ☐   C   Tension pneumothorax
   ☐   D   Left-sided pleural effusion
   ☐   E   Mediastinitis.

Answer overleaf   **Case 1**

Answer

     1   C   **Tension pneumothorax.**

Discussion

This patient developed a tension pneumothorax immediately after the laser therapy due to perforation of the tumour through into the right pleural space. There is complete collapse of the right lung and the pleural space is full of air. The right hemithorax is more radiolucent than the left. The right hemidiaphragm is depressed compared with the normal position of the left hemidiaphragm.

There is also shift of the mediastinum over to the left and within the mediastinum there are linear streaks of air representing mediastinal emphysema. The left lung remains expanded and there is no evidence of sub-diaphragmatic air.

Tension pneumothorax is potentially life threatening and occurs when the intrapleural pressure is high enough to compress the lung. The damage to the lung results in a tear which acts as a flap valve.

The shift of the mediastinum to the other side and the depression of the hemidiaphragm are the most important radiological signs. In this case, however, the right lung itself was not damaged but the pneumothorax was probably related to air insufflation through the endoscope.

The presence of mediastinal emphysema in this case is as a result of the oesophageal perforation and is not a usual feature of a tension pneumothorax.

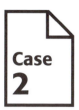

Case 2

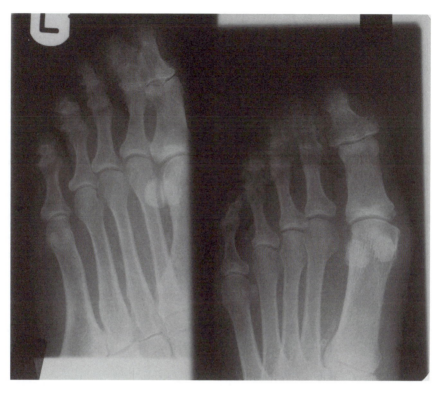

A 76-year-old man is diabetic and suffers from increasing pain in the foot.

Question

2   What is the most likely diagnosis? See also Case 113.
- ☐ A   Gout
- ☐ B   Osteomyelitis
- ☐ C   Peripheral vascular disease with vascular calcification
- ☐ D   Gangrenous big toe.

Answer overleaf   Case 2

Answer

2 B **Osteomyelitis.**

Discussion

At the base of the terminal phalanx of the second toe there is an area where the bone has been destroyed. There is little in the way of periosteal reaction associated with this, however. In addition there is marked calcification of the metatarsal arteries which is a common finding in patients with diabetes.

This calcification in the vessels does not necessarily imply that there is significant peripheral vascular disease although this is frequently present in diabetes. The bony destruction of the base of the terminal phalanx is consistent with infection in the bone and surrounding soft tissues.

In diabetes a peripheral neuropathy combined with a degree of vascular insufficiency may lead to ulceration and secondary infection is not uncommon.

In gout soft tissue masses due to tophi may be seen adjacent to the joint and erosions tend to be away from the joint margin, often affecting both sides of the joint.

The articular cartilage is lost late in the disease process. When a toe becomes gangrenous air may be seen within the soft tissues.

Case 3

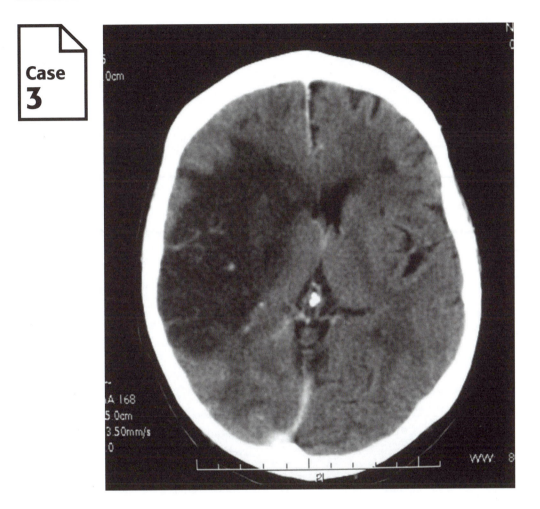

This is the enhanced CT brain scan of a 70-year-old man who presented with a left hemiplegia.

Question

3   What is the most likely diagnosis?

☐   A   Intracerebral bleed
☐   B   Malignant glioma
☐   C   Right cerebral infarction
☐   D   Subdural haematoma
☐   E   Metastasis from primary bronchial carcinoma.

Answer overleaf

Answer

    3   C   **Right cerebral infarction.**

Discussion

This is a contrast enhanced CT scan of the brain and shows a well demarcated area of low density in the right cerebral hemisphere. There is mass effect with obliteration of the anterior horn of the right lateral ventricle and there is a slight degree of displacement of the third ventricle (a midline structure) to the left. There is also obliteration of the right Sylvian fissure.

In the investigation of an acute cerebrovascular event intravenous contrast enhancement is not necessary to distinguish between a cerebral bleed and cerebral infarction. The distribution of the low density change here is in the territory supplied by the middle cerebral artery and is consistent with a right middle cerebral artery occlusion. The mass effect is due to oedema of the infarcted brain.

Within the area of infarction the right middle cerebral artery can be seen as a higher density structure since it is enhanced by contrast medium. In an acute thrombosis of a cerebral vessel, the thrombus within the vessel may produce a high density (in the absence of intravenous contrast medium).

This patient had been given intravenous contrast in order to exclude an underlying metastasis. A metastasis would typically appear as an enhancing lesion with surrounding oedema. Irregular enhancement within the area of low density would be expected if this lesion were a malignant glioma and a malignant tumour would not be as clearly demarcated and confined to the middle cerebral artery territory.

There is no evidence here of any fresh blood within the brain, dural spaces or subarachnoid space. In an acute haemorrhage fresh blood is of high density.

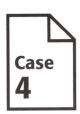

Case
4

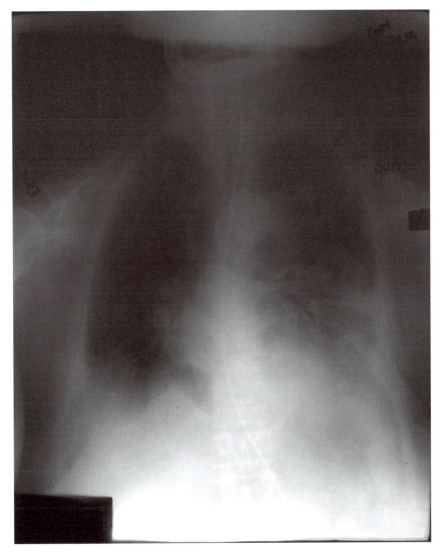

This 85-year-old woman who was being fed via a nasogastric tube developed acute shortness of breath.

Question

4   What is the most likely diagnosis?
- [ ]   A   Left lower lobe consolidation
- [ ]   B   Left lower lobe collapse
- [ ]   C   Right side haemothorax
- [ ]   D   Pulmonary oedema.

Answer overleaf

Case
4

Answer

4   A   **Left lower lobe consolidation.**

Discussion

Within the left lower zone an air bronchogram is clearly visible. In the normal patient the main airways may be seen in the lung as far out as the main bronchi. Segmental bronchi are not usually seen in the normal lung except when seen end on.

An air bronchogram is seen where bronchi are passing through lung parenchyma that is no longer aerated but filled with secretions or inflammatory debris. An air bronchogram is most commonly seen in pneumonias although it may be observed in pulmonary oedema.

In this patient the air bronchogram is confined to the left lower lobe. There is no significant volume loss associated with this to suggest the presence of left lower lobe collapse.

This patient does have bilateral pleural effusions in addition but there are no other signs of cardiac failure such as upper zone blood diversion.

Case
5

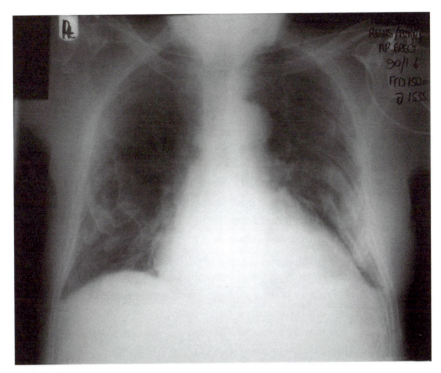

This 79-year-old man presents with a myocardial infarction.

Question

5   What is seen on the chest x-ray?
  ☐   A   Pulmonary oedema
  ☐   B   Asbestos pleural plaques
  ☐   C   Asbestosis
  ☐   D   Old calcified empyema
  ☐   E   Mesothelioma.

Answer overleaf

Case
5

Answer

5 B **Asbestos pleural plaques.**

Discussion

There is extensive pleural calicification on both sides of the chest in this patient. These are typical of asbestos-related pleural plaques. They are usually more prominent in the lower half of the thorax and they may follow the rib contours and may also be seen on the surface of the diaphragm. They are usually bilateral and the apices are usually spared.

Pleural plaques from asbestos exposure appear more than 20 years after exposure to asbestos. They are on the parietal pleura. Where plaques are seen in profile the calcification is seen as linear and when seen en-face have the appearance often described as holly-leaf. Pleural plaques do not themselves change into malignant mesothelioma although plaques may be present in patients with mesothelioma.

Mesothelioma typically consists of extensive nodular thickening of the pleural and is usually unlilateral. The pleural thickening may encase the whole of a lung and extend into the fissures. It is usually associated with a pleural effusion and there is often volume loss of the hemithorax.

Asbestos plaques are distinct from asbestosis which is the interstitial fibrosis due to asbestos.

Pleural calcification from an old empyema is usually much more sheet-like and associated with more marked pleural thickening which may result in the pleural calcification separated from the margins of the hemithorax.

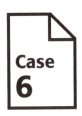

Case
6

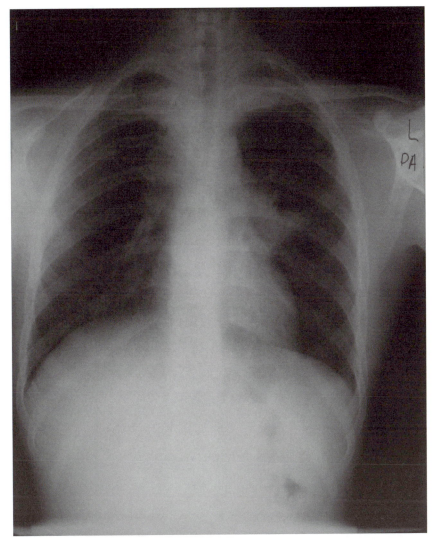

This 24-year-old man has a dry cough and night sweats.

Question

6   What is the most likely diagnosis?

☐   A   Sarcoidosis
☐   B   Tuberculosis
☐   C   Mitral valve disease
☐   D   Pulmonary hypertension
☐   E   Aortic aneurysm.

Answer overleaf   Case
6

Answer

6   B   **Tuberculosis.**

Discussion

There is left hilar lymphadenopathy and also right paratracheal lymphadenopathy. There is also filling in of the aorto-pulmonary window on the left due to adenopathy here.

The right hilum itself is spared of lymphadenopathy and this would be unusual in the case of sarcoidosis.

In pulmonary hypertension the proximal pulmonary arteries are enlarged but there should be symmetrical enlargement of both hilar.

With mitral valve disease there may be enlargement of the left atrial appendage, which is seen as a third convexity beneath the main pulmonary outflow tract.

In this patient the upper part of the left heart border may be seen distinct from the lymphadenopathy. The right paratracheal lymphadenopathy extends too high for this to be an aneurysm of the ascending aorta.

This proved to be tuberculosis with predominant nodal disease rather than parenchymal disease.

Case 7

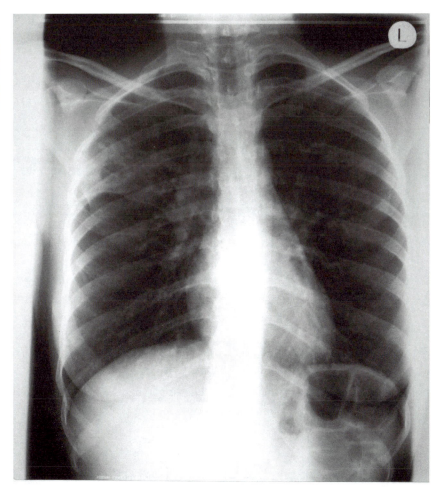

This 33-year-old woman presents with a dry cough and loss of weight.

Question

7 What is the most likely diagnosis?
- ☐ A Lobar pneumonia of the right upper lobe
- ☐ B Right upper lobe tuberculosis
- ☐ C Right upper lobe collapse
- ☐ D Right paratracheal lymphadenopathy.

Answer overleaf

Case 7

Answer

    7 B   **Right upper lobe tuberculosis.**

Discussion

There is patchy consolidation in the right upper lobe and there is elevation of the horizontal fissure on the right indicating a degree of volume loss in the right upper lobe. There is also cavitation seen within the lower part of the right upper lobe.

There is no evidence of any paratracheal lymphadenopathy. The combination of volume loss consolidation and cavitation is very suspicious of tuberculosis. The patient had tubercle bacilli identified in a sputum smear.

A lobar pneumonia in the right upper lobe may produce patchy consolidation like this although usually produces a much more confluent pattern of consolidation. Bronchopneumonia uncommonly is confined to an upper lobe.

The paratracheal regions are normal and there is no evidence here of any hilar or paratracheal lymphadenopathy.

Although the horizontal fissure is slightly elevated, this should not be visible if there had been complete right upper lobe collapse.

Case 8

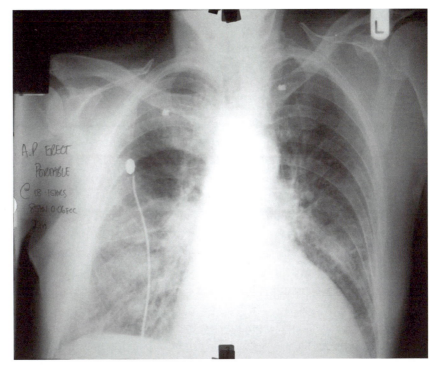

This 67-year-old man presents with chest pain and shortness of breath.

Question

8   What is the most likely diagnosis?
- ☐   A   Bronchial pneumonia
- ☐   B   Pulmonary oedema
- ☐   C   Pneumocystis pneumonia
- ☐   D   Lymphangitis carcinomatosis.

Answer overleaf

Answer

8   B   **Pulmonary oedema.**

Discussion

This is an AP (antero-posterior) film which does tend to make the heart look larger than a conventional PA film. There is prominence of the pulmonary vessels and diffuse interstitial shadowing extending out from both hila into the lung fields. Some septal lines are seen and there is thickening of the horizontal fissure on the right. There is lack of clarity of the intra-pulmonary vessels and frank alveolar oedema in the right lower zone.

Bat's wing and butterfly shadowing are terms used to describe this perihilar shadowing which is predominantly central and tends to spare the periphery of the lung. The classic bat's wing pattern is relatively uncommon, however.

In bronchial pneumonia there is usually patchy consolidation and the pulmonary vessels should not be as prominent as here.

In lymphangitis carcinomatosis there may be pleural thickening due to sub-pleural oedema but the interstitial shadowing is more reticulonodular than that seen here. In addition septal lines may also be seen and there are often bilateral pleural effusions.

Pneumocystis carinii pneumonia typically has fine perihilar reticular shadowing and there may be an ill-defined ground-glass appearance but the pulmonary vessels are not as prominent as here.

Case
8

Case 9

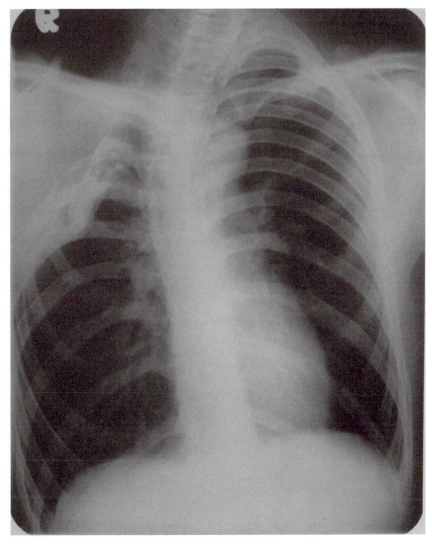

This 68-year-old man is under regular follow-up at the chest clinic.

Question

9   What is the most likely diagnosis?
- [ ] A   Right upper lobectomy
- [ ] B   Right thoracoplasty
- [ ] C   Apical plombage
- [ ] D   Congenital scoliosis.

Answer overleaf

Case 9

Answer

9 B **Right thoracoplasty.**

Discussion

The right first to fifth ribs have been resected and the right upper lobe has collapsed down. The film below (Figure 9A) shows the chest radiograph at the time of diagnosis 50 years previously. There is extensive nodulation and cavitation in the right upper lobe consistent with tuberculosis.

Thoracoplasty was employed in the treatment of tuberculosis and consisted of resection of a number of ribs to collapse the chest wall down onto the lung.

In some cases this was so extensive that only a little lung was left at the base. Thoracoplasty was employed along with other techniques to collapse the lung such as apical plombage with Lucite balls and artificial pneumothorax in the management of tuberculosis.

This patient has developed a scoliosis secondary to the rib resections.

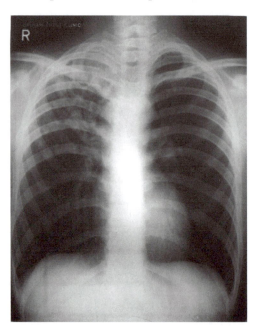

Figure 9A

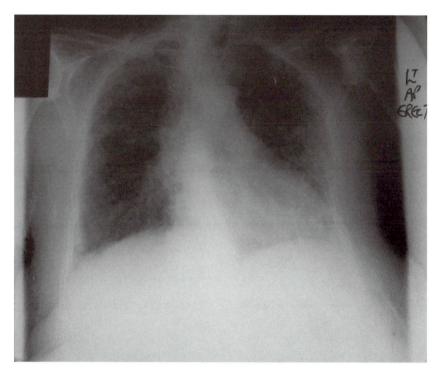

An 88-year-old lady presents with shortness of breath.

Question

10 What is the most likely diagnosis?
- ☐ A   Sarcoidosis
- ☐ B   Miliary tuberculosis
- ☐ C   Miliary metastases
- ☐ D   Bronchial pneumonia
- ☐ E   Pulmonary oedema.

Answer overleaf

Answer

10   C   **Miliary metastases.**

Discussion

This film shows multiple nodules ranging in size from 2–3 mm extending throughout the whole of both lungs. This may be described as miliary shadowing.

There is a wide differential diagnosis for miliary nodules:
Miliary tuberculosis
Other infections:
- histoplasmosis
- nocardiosis
- blastomycosis
- cryptococcosis
Pneumoconiosis
Sarcoidosis
Miliary metastases:
- most commonly thyroid, renal carcinoma and melanoma
Alveolar microlithiasis.

There is no evidence of any hilar lymphadenopathy in this patient to suggest sarcoidosis and there was no occupational history to suggest a pneumoconiosis.

It is not possible to exclude miliary tuberculosis in this patient. Other infections such as histoplasmosis are almost unknown in the UK.

The differential diagnosis in this case was between miliary metastases and miliary tuberculosis. The patient died fairly soon after admission and at post-mortem the patient was found to have multiple pulmonary metastases from a primary endometrial carcinoma.

Case
10

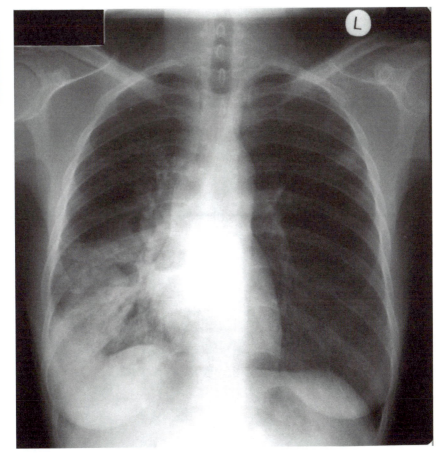

A 36-year-old lady presented with cough and weight loss.

Question

11   What is the most likely diagnosis?
- ☐ **A** Right lower lobe collapse
- ☐ **B** Right lower lobe tuberculosis
- ☐ **C** Pulmonary infarction.

Answer overleaf

Answer

11   B   **Right lower lobe tuberculosis**.

Discussion

There is extensive consolidation in the right lower zone, which shows
evidence of cavitation. The CT scan (Figure 11A), which was carried out,
clearly showed large cavitating lesions in the right lower lobe and also some
consolidation in the right middle lobe. There is also a small right-sided
pleural effusion. There is a little volume loss as evidenced by a slightly low
horizontal fissure, but the main feature is consolidation rather than collapse.
The extensive cavitation and pleural fluid is highly suspicious of tuberculosis
and the patient was proven to be smear positive for tubercle bacilli.
Pulmonary infarction can also cavitate but there were no predisposing
factors in this case.

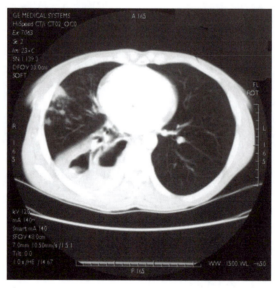

Figure 11A

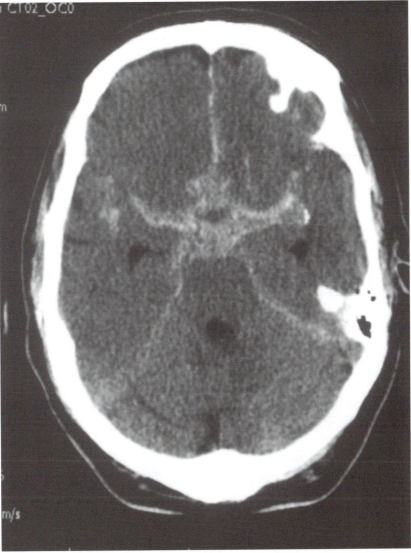

This 70-year-old woman presented with sudden onset of headache then loss of consciousness.

Question

12   What is the most likely diagnosis?
- ☐ A   Stroke secondary to infarction
- ☐ B   Acute extradural haemorrhage
- ☐ C   Acute subdural haemorrhage
- ☐ D   Acute subarachnoid haemorrhage.

Answer overleaf

Answer

    12   D   **Acute subarachnoid haemorrhage**.

Discussion

On this unenhanced CT of the brain there is high attenuation material in the subarachnoid space surrounding the Circle of Willis. In this patient, the haemorrhage was secondary to a ruptured aneurysm of the right posterior communicating artery.

Case
12

Case 13

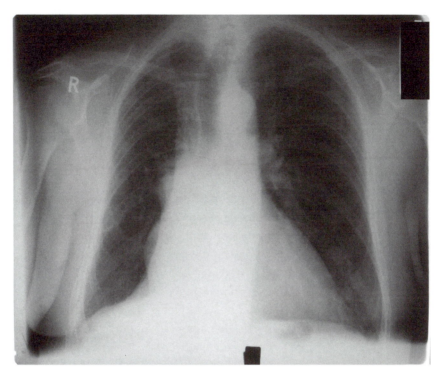

This 83-year-old man presents with weight loss and cough.

Question

13   What is the most likely diagnosis?
- [ ] A   Right lower lobe pneumonia
- [ ] B   Right lower lobe collapse
- [ ] C   Right upper lobe collapse
- [ ] D   Right middle lobe pneumonia
- [ ] E   Right middle lobe collapse.

Answer overleaf

Case 13

Answer

13   B   **Right lower lobe collapse.**

Discussion

On the right side there is a triangular opacity based on the diaphragm and the mediastinum representing a collapsed right lower lobe. When the right lower lobe collapses completely it comes to lie posteromedially in the lower part of the chest.

A right lower lobe collapse is more easily recognised than a left lower lobe collapse which may be obscured by the heart. The right hemithorax is overall slightly smaller than the left hemithorax. The right middle and upper lobes over-expand to fill the space vacated by the collapsed lobe and the pulmonary vessels in these lobes becomes wider apart. Along with the collapsed lobe the inferior pulmonary lobe vessels are no longer visible.

The most common cause of lobar atelectasis or collapse is a bronchial obstruction due to either a tumour or a mucous plug. Inhaled foreign bodies are less common in adults than children. Occasionally enlarged hilar nodes can result in a lobar collapse.

In this patient bronchoscopy revealed a carcinoma in the right lower lobe bronchus.

Right upper lobe collapse results in the lobe moving towards the upper part of the mediastinum and the middle and lower lobes over-expand and the right basal pulmonary vessels are displaced upwards and outwards.

Right middle lobe collapse can be very difficult to detect since it may be too thin to see but loss of the silhouette of the right heart border is the major feature.

See also Case 65 (lobar collapse).

Case
13

Case
14

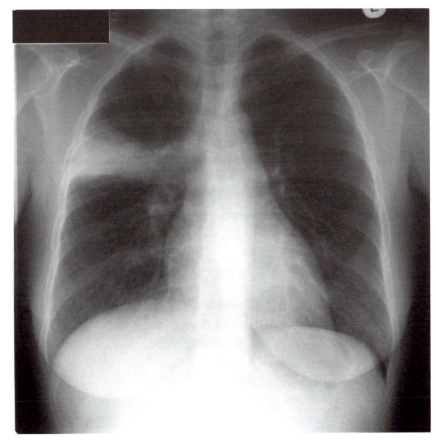

This 34-year-old woman has a cough, pyrexia and dull right-sided chest pain.

Question

14   What is the most likely diagnosis?

- ☐ **A**   Right upper lobe pneumonia
- ☐ **B**   Bronchial pneumonia
- ☐ **C**   Aspiration pneumonia
- ☐ **D**   Pulmonary embolus.

Answer overleaf

Case
14

Answer

14 A **Right upper lobe pneumonia.**

Discussion

In the right upper lobe there is a clearly demarcated area of increased density which is sharply limited on the inferior aspect by the horizontal fissure. This is consolidation in the anterior segment of the right upper lobe. The straight lower margin of this area is a gravitational effect with the debris in the alveoli sinking to the most dependent part of the segment which is limited by the horizontal fissure.

An air bronchogram may be seen in consolidated lung but here the consolidation is quite peripheral in the segment and bronchi cannot be identified. The most likely cause for lobar consolidation such as this is a lobar pneumonia.

It is unlikely that aspiration pneumonia would affect the anterior segment of the right upper lobe and aspiration is more usually seen in the lower lobes.

Bronchial pneumonia is not usually as clearly demarcated as this consolidation and the consolidation tends to be more patchy and may not be confined to one lobe or segment.

Pulmonary infarcts may produce a segmental consolidation but would be expected to have a better defined upper margin than is seen here.

Case **15**

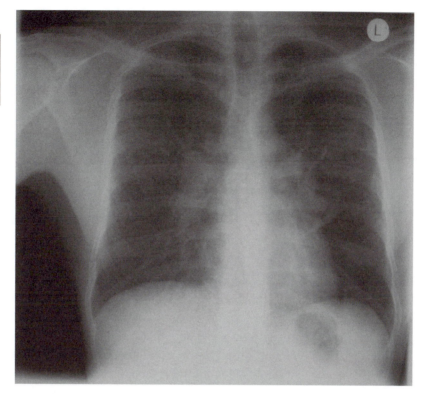

This is a 30-year-old man with a dry cough.

Question

15   What is the most likely diagnosis?
- ☐ A   Miliary tuberculosis
- ☐ B   Miliary metastases
- ☐ C   Sarcoidosis
- ☐ D   Lymphoma.

Answer overleaf

Case **15**

Answer

15   C   **Sarcoidosis.**

Discussion

Both hila are enlarged due to lymphadenopathy and there is extensive nodular shadowing ranging from 2–3 mm throughout both lungs.

Hilar lymphadenopathy produces overall enlargement of the hilum and a lobulated outline and there may be a rounded mass of tissue in an area where there are no normal vascular structures such as between the aortic arch and the pulmonary outflow tract: the aorto-pulmonary window.

In this case there is also a rounded mass in between the right upper and lower lobe vessels. There is no paratracheal lymphadenopathy which would be unusual if this were lymphoma.

Fine nodules such as seen in the lungs here may be described as miliary nodules and there are many causes (see Case 10). The combination in this case of the large hilar nodes and miliary nodules is typical of sarcoidosis.

Miliary tuberculosis may have nodules like this but the hilar lymphadenopathy is too florid for miliary tuberculosis. This pattern is also very unusual for miliary metastases with hilar node involvement as well.

Case
15

Case
16

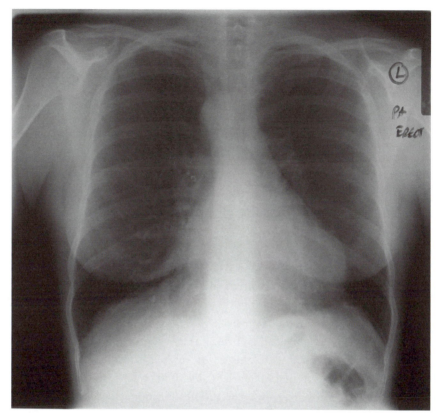

This 33-year-old woman presents with hypertension.

Question

16   What is the most likely diagnosis?

☐   A   Coarctation of the aorta

☐   B   Marfan's syndrome

☐   C   Paratracheal lymphadenopathy

☐   D   Right-sided aortic arch.

Answer overleaf

Case
16

Answer

16   D   **Right-sided aortic arch.**

Discussion

There is a smooth mass-like abnormality to the right of the trachea in the upper mediastinum and the trachea is displaced slightly to the left. On the left side of the mediastinum there is no aortic knuckle visible above the pulmonary outflow tract. This is a right sided aortic arch.

A right sided aortic arch may have mirror image branches and is usually associated with cyanotic congenital heart disease.

A right sided arch with an aberrant left subclavian artery occurs in 0.1% of the population. In this instance the first branch of the aorta is the left common carotid artery followed by the right common carotid artery, the right subclavian artery and the left subclavian artery. The left subclavian artery is aberrant in that it passes posterior to the oesophagus before it passes up onto the neck.

A right sided arch such as this is usually asymptomatic and is not associated with other cardiovascular abnormalities. The right sided arch tends to indent the right side of the trachea and may be slightly higher than a normal left-sided arch. The descending aorta is usually in the right posterior mediastinum and rarely descends on the left of the mediastinum.

Case 16

Case
17

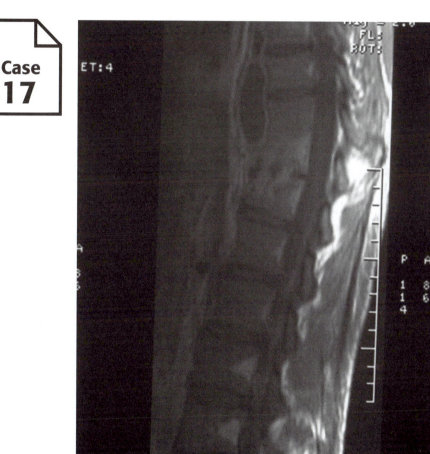

This 34-year-old man has persistent pain in the right hip and upper thigh.

Question

17   What is the most likely diagnosis?

☐   A   Metastatic disease to vertebral bodies

☐   B   Meningomyelocoele

☐   C   Infective discitis

☐   D   Prolapsed intervertebral disc.

Answer overleaf

Case
17

Answer

17   C   **Infective discitis.**

Discussion

This is a T1-weighted gadolinium enhanced sagittal magnetic resonance image of the lower spine. The vertebra are seen as low signal strips of cortical bone surrounding higher signal cancellous bone which is best seen in the upper vertebrae in this case.

The normal intervertebral discs are seen with a central darker area (the nucleus pulposus with a higher water content). The triangular-shaped area of high signal in the posterior aspect of the vertebral bodies represents the basivertebral vein complex. In the spinal canal the cord and cauda equina are clearly seen due to the low signal of CSF on T1-weighted images.

There is an acute kyphosis at T11 and the discs at T10–11 and T11–12 have lost their normal signal characteristics and are partially destroyed. They are replaced by soft tissue which has enhanced abnormally.

The signal in the adjacent vertebral bodies is abnormal with loss of the basivertebral vein complex. In addition there is a paravertebral fluid collection which has a thick enhancing rim and was shown to extend from T7 down to T12.

More inferiorly fluid collections of similar signal characteristics extended into the psoas muscles on either side. These appearances are in keeping with tuberculous discitis and associated osteomyelitis and psoas abscess formation.

Disc space infections may be accompanied by osteomyelitis in the adjacent vertebral bodies which may be compressed. The infectious process may extend into the soft tissues in the paravertebral regions and may also extend into the epidural space forming an epidural abscess. This has not happened in this case, however.

Case
17

Case 18

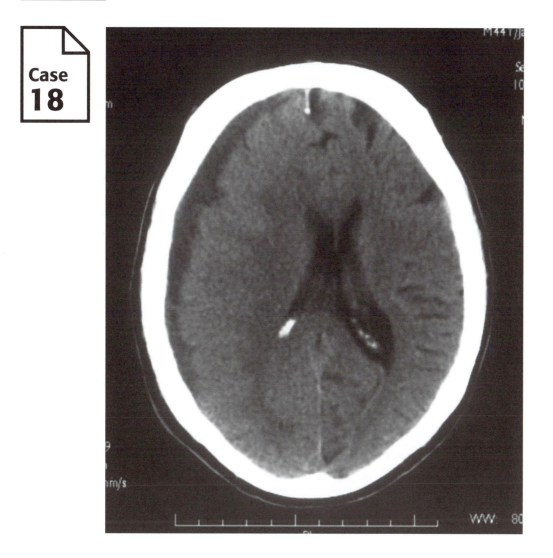

An unenchanced CT scan in a 44-year-old man presenting with increasing confusion.

Question

18   What is the most likely diagnosis?

☐   A   Acute subdural haemorrhage

☐   B   Acute extradural haemorrhage

☐   C   Chronic subdural haemorrhage

☐   D   Chronic extradural haemorrhage.

Answer overleaf   Case 18

Answer

18   C   **Chronic subdural haemorrhage.**

Discussion

This is an unenhanced CT scan. On the right side of the brain there is a rim of low-density material which surrounds the right cerebral hemisphere. There is effacement of the cerebral sulci and a degree of mid-line shift to the left. This low density material is a chronic subdural haematoma.

In the normal state the vascular structures in the brain are of the same density as the brain. In an acute cerebral haemorrhage the blood which has left the confines of vessels is still the same density as the brain substance but once there is resorption of some of the fluid content it becomes high attenuation.

An acute evolving haematoma becomes of higher density than normal brain. Without intervention, in time the protein density of a haematoma becomes less and the haematoma will go through a phase of being isodense with brain. This may occur between 7 and 21 days after the acute episode.

Further absorption of protein results in a chronic haematoma which is of lower density compared to normal brain and eventually has a similar density to cerebrospinal fluid.

An extradural haemorrhage is usually caused by trauma and the haematoma is confined by the dura mater which is firmly attached to the cranial sutures. An extradural haematoma will not cross suture lines. A subdural haematoma, however, collects in the potential space between the dura mater and the arachnoid mater and as it is not confined by the sutures can spread over the surface of the brain to produce the concave shaped inner margin as seen here.

See also Case 47.

Case
18

Case 19

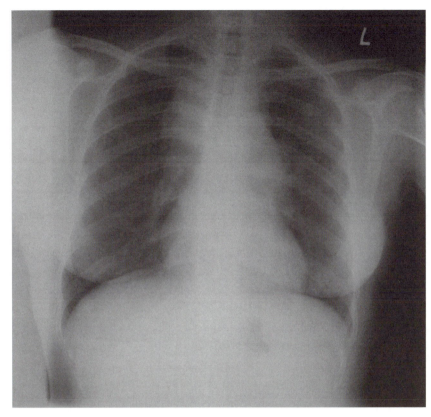

This 45-year-old patient has a cough and loss of weight.

Question

19   What is the most likely diagnosis?
  - ☐   A   Lymphoma
  - ☐   B   Tuberculous lymphadenopathy
  - ☐   C   Metastatic breast cancer
  - ☐   D   Sarcoidosis.

Answer overleaf

Case 19

Answer

19   B   **Tuberculous lymphadenopathy**.

Discussion

There is a large right paratracheal mass and there is also lymphadenopathy in the aorto-pulmonary window on the left. The carina is also splayed by some subcarinal lymphadenopathy.

Within the mid and upper zones of the left lung are some areas of calcification which are consistent with old granulomas caused by tuberculosis. There is also destruction of a portion of the left 4th rib.

The asymmetry of the hilar and paratracheal adenopathy would be unusual for sarcoidosis and there are no pulmonary nodules, although lack of pulmonary involvement does not exclude sarcoidosis.

Lymphoma needs to be considered in the differential diagnosis although again the asymmetrical nature of the adenopathy would be unusual.

The rib destruction could be due to metastatic disease but in metastatic breast cancer it would be unusual to see this degree of lymphadenopathy without pulmonary metastases.

Rib involvement in sarcoidosis is exceedingly rare and very few cases have been described. Osteitis with rib destruction however is a recognised thoracic complication of tuberculosis.

This patient was proven to have tuberculosis.

Case
19

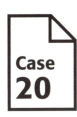

Case
20

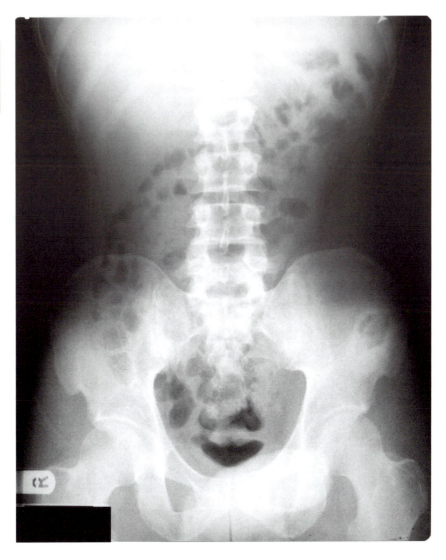

This 46-year-old man has a pain in the left hip.

Question

20   What is the most likely diagnosis?
  ☐   A   Psoas abscess with involvement of the iliac wing
  ☐   B   Metastasis in the left iliac wing
  ☐   C   Sacroiliitis
  ☐   D   Septic arthritis of the left hip.

Answer overleaf

Case
20

Answer

20   A   **Psoas abscess with involvement of the iliac wing.**

Discussion

The abdominal film shows that neither of the psoas margins are clearly seen. There is a lucent defect in the left iliac wing with a slightly sclerotic margin. The sacro-iliac joints are normal and both hip joints are also normal. A CT scan (Figure 20A) showed a large fluid collection replacing the left psoas muscle and on bony windows (Figure 20B) a destructive lesion in the left iliac wing was clearly delineated. Aspiration of the psoas abscess revealed tubercle bacilli. This was a tuberculous psoas abscess with associated osteomyelitis of the iliac wing.

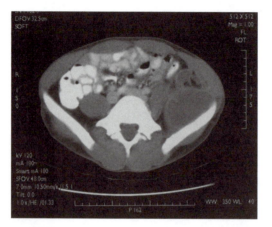

Figure 20A

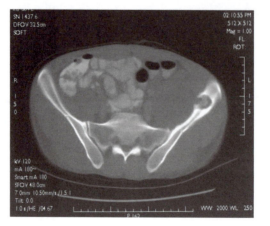

Figure 20B

Case
20

Case
21

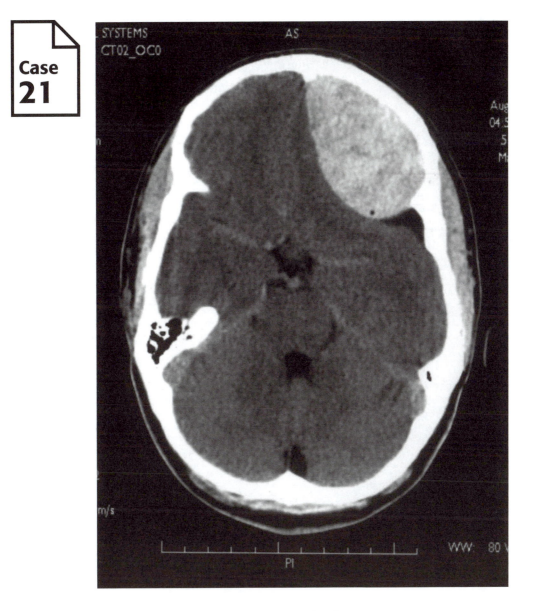

This 22-year-old man presented with a head injury.

Question

21   What is the most likely diagnosis?

☐ A   Chronic extradural haemorrhage
☐ B   Acute extradural haemorrhage
☐ C   Chronic subdural haemorrhage
☐ D   Acute subdural haemorrhage.

Answer overleaf

Case
21

Answer

21   B   **Acute extradural haemorrhage**.

Discussion

This unenhanced CT scan of the brain shows a high-density collection in the anterior cranial fossa. There is quite marked compression and distortion of the left frontal lobe and there is some midline shift to the right side. This high density material is fresh blood.

The inner margin is convex and it is limited by the attachment of the dura mater to the frontal bone and the coronal suture. This is a neurosurgical emergency.

Subdural haematomas are not contained by the attachments of the dural and spread around the surface of the brain much more easily.

With time, if left untreated, an acute haematoma will pass through a phase of being iso-dense with brain substance as the haemoglobin content and protein content is absorbed. Eventually a haematoma will become of low density resembling the density of cerebrospinal fluid when it has become a chronic haematoma.

Most extradural haematomas as in this case are the result of trauma often with involvement of the middle meningeal artery.

Case
21

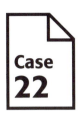

Case 22

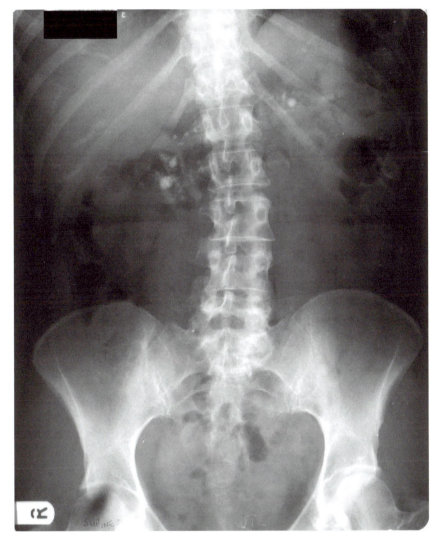

This 64-year-old lady has a long-standing history of epigastric pain.

Question

22   What is the most likely diagnosis?
- ☐ A   Chronic pancreatitis
- ☐ B   Acute pancreatitis
- ☐ C   Adenocarcinoma of the pancreas
- ☐ D   Calcified mesenteric lymph nodes
- ☐ E   Chronic calcific pancreatitis.

Answer overleaf

Case 22

Answer

22   E   **Chronic calcific pancreatitis.**

Discussion

This plain abdominal film shows punctate calcification in the upper abdomen which extends from the right side lateral to the right side of the 2nd lumbar vertebra across the midline and up in the left upper quadrant. This punctate calcification is typical of chronic calcific pancreatitis.

The calcification represents calcified filling defects within a dilated main pancreatic duct and within dilated side branches. Calcific pancreatitis like this is highly suggestive of alcohol-related pancreatitis.

Chronic pancreatitis can occur without the presence of calcification in the ducts. In chronic pancreatitis the size of the pancreas is very variable. The gland can become atrophic from chronic inflammation and fibrosis but can also be enlarged either uniformly or focally.

An acute exacerbation of chronic pancreatitis cannot be entirely excluded although in this case there is no evidence of small bowel distention (the sentinel loop).

Adenocarcinoma of the pancreas can occur in patients with chronic pancreatitis but the primary tumour does not usually calcify.

Although calcified mesenteric lymph nodes are frequently seen the distribution of the calcification in this patient is typical of pancreatic calcification.

Case
22

Case 23

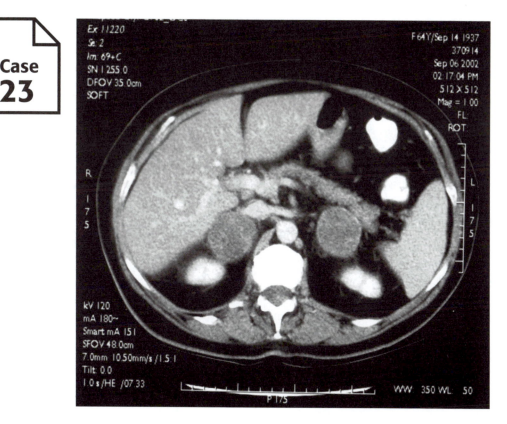

This 64-year-old lady has a six-month oncology follow-up.

Question

23   What is the most likely diagnosis?
- ☐   A   Renal cysts
- ☐   B   Adrenal cysts
- ☐   C   Phaeochromocytomas
- ☐   D   Bilateral adrenal metastases.

Answer overleaf   **Case 23**

Answer

23   D   **Bilateral adrenal metastases.**

Discussion

This contrast enhanced CT scan of the upper abdomen shows two discrete masses anterior to the kidneys with a rim of enhancement. They are not of fluid density, are separate from the kidneys and are not renal cysts.

These are in the position of the adrenal glands and represent bilateral adrenal metastases. The patient had a history of melanoma and the adrenal gland is a recognised site for melanoma metastases.

Unilateral adrenal metastases are more common than bilateral metastases. Common sites of origin are melanoma, kidney, breast and lung. They usually have an enhancing rim following iv contrast medium.

Phaeochromocytomas can be bilateral in up to 10% of cases. They tend to be in excess of 5 cm diameter and show intense contrast enhancement.

Adrenocortical adenomas and non-functioning adenomas contain areas of fat density on CT.

Case
23

Case
24

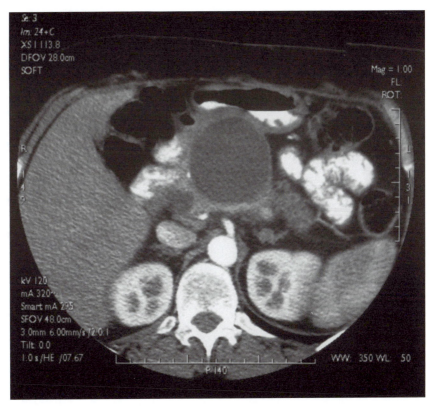

This is a 48-year-old woman with chronic epigastric discomfort.

Question

24   What is the most likely diagnosis?

☐ A   Pancreatic pseudocysts

☐ B   Acute pancreatitis

☐ C   Gastrointestinal stromal tumour (GIST).

Answer overleaf

Case
24

Answer

24   A   **Pancreatic pseudocysts.**

Discussion

This contrast enhanced CT of the abdomen shows a well circumscribed 5 cm fluid collection. This is lying separate from and posterior to the stomach. There is a fleck of calcification in the wall of the lesion and there is a further smaller fluid collection within the head of the pancreas.

There are no inflammatory changes in the adjacent mesentery and no evidence of free intraperitoneal fluid. The tail of the pancreas is of normal size and does not contain any calcification. The appearance of this fluid collection is consistent with a pancreatic pseudocyst.

Pancreatic pseudocysts evolve from acute fluid collections at the time of an attack of acute pancreatitis and take a few weeks to fully evolve into discrete cysts with a fibrous capsule or wall. Up to 50% of pancreatic pseudocysts resolve spontaneously.

Gastrointestinal stromal tumours (GIST) includes what were previously regarded as leiomyomas and 70% of them occur in the stomach. They arise within the wall of the stomach and in this case the lesion is clearly seen separate from the stomach. They are usually of soft tissue density and enhance to a variable degree following intravenous contrast medium.

Case 25

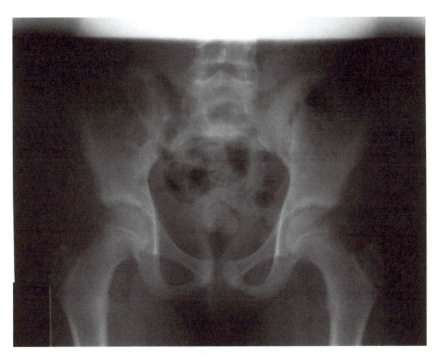

This 13-year-old girl presents with painful hips and knees.

Question

25   What is the most likely diagnosis?
- ☐ **A** Scurvy
- ☐ **B** Slipped femoral epiphysis
- ☐ **C** Septic arthritis
- ☐ **D** Vitamin D deficiency rickets.

Answer overleaf

Case 25

Answer

25   D   **Vitamin D deficiency rickets.**

Discussion

This AP pelvis shows quite marked widening of the epiphyses of the greater trochanters of both femora with some subchondral sclerosis. In vitamin D deficiency rickets recently formed bone at the growth plate does not become calcified resulting in apparent widening of the growth plate. These changes are found at the more rapidly growing bone ends.

There is an increased distance across the epiphysis followed by splaying and cupping of the metaphysis. This is seen typically in the distal radius. This girl has developed rickets at the start of her pre-pubertal growth spurt.

The femoral head epiphyses are also slightly widened but the position of the femoral head in relation to the femoral metaphysis is normal.

Slipped femoral epiphysis occurs between the ages of 10 and 15 years and usually presents as a limp. It may be bilateral in 20–40% of cases. The femoral epiphysis slips posteriorly and medially and results in lateral displacement of the femoral metaphysis in relation to the medial margin of the acetabulum.

In cases of septic arthritis there is an increase in the joint space due to a joint effusion and there may be osteopaenia of the surrounding bone. Rapid and progressive destruction of articular cartilage may occur.

Case
25

Case
26

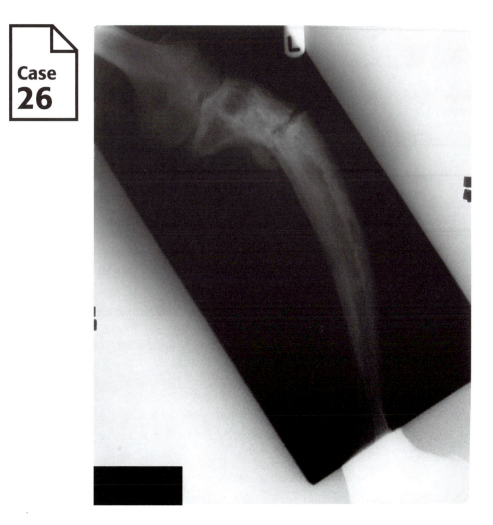

This 82-year-old man has difficulty walking.

Question

26 What is the most likely diagnosis?
- ☐ A Paget's disease with a stress fracture
- ☐ B Metastases from prostatic carcinoma
- ☐ C Chronic osteomyelitis.

Answer overleaf **Case 26**

Answer

26 A **Paget's disease with a pathological fracture.**

Discussion

This lateral view of the tibia shows considerable bowing of the shaft of the tibia and a fracture through the upper metaphysis. The bony texture of the tibia is very abnormal with a coarse trabecular pattern. The abnormality extends up to the articular surface of the tibia at the knee. The appearances are of a pathological fracture through the tibia involved by Paget's disease.

Paget's disease shows three distinct radiological appearances which may all be present within affected bones:
• Predominantly lytic disease as is seen in osteoporosis circumscripta in the skull
• New bone growing from the cortex into the medulla resulting in enlargement of the bone and a coarse trabecular pattern
• Diffuse increase in density with bone enlargement.

Complications of Paget's disease are not uncommon:
• Marginal fractures on an abnormal convex surface
• Spontaneous fractures such as in the humerus
• Osteoarthritis where joint surfaces are involved
• Development of osteosarcoma.

Bony metastases from prostate carcinoma are usually sclerotic and may be either discrete areas of sclerosis or more diffuse confluent metastases.

In chronic osteomyelitis there is often abnormal modelling of bone and quite marked sclerosis. There may be a cavity containing a sequestrum with surrounding sclerosis.

Case 27

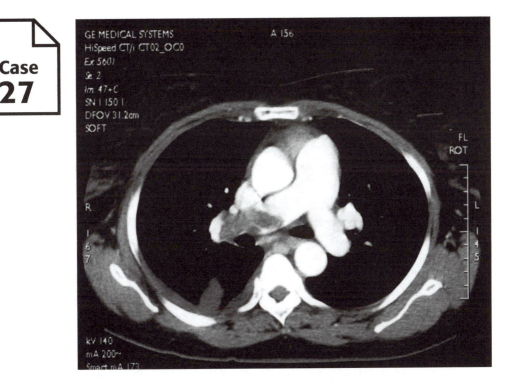

A 55-year-old woman with central chest pain and breathlessness.

Question

27   What is the most likely diagnosis?

   ☐   **A**   Bronchial carcinoma.

   ☐   **B**   Hilar lymphadenopathy

   ☐   **C**   Pulmonary embolus.

Answer overleaf

Case **27**

Answer

27   C   **Pulmonary embolus**.

Discussion

This is a CT pulmonary angiogram. The patient has been given an intravenous bolus of contrast medium and the scan timed so that the maximum concentration of contrast is in the pulmonary arteries at the time of scanning.

Within the right main pulmonary artery there is a large lobulated filling defect which is due to a large embolus lodged in the vessel. Central pulmonary emboli like this are likely to remain for up to several weeks. More peripheral emboli which can be detected on CT pulmonary angiography may disappear within a few days after commencement of anticoagulation. CT pulmonary angiography is recommended in patients with equivocal ventilation/perfusion scans.

Additionally there is a pleurally-based soft tissue density in the posterior segment of the right upper lobe consistent with a pulmonary infarction. There is no evidence on this image of hilar mass nor of an intrapulmonary mass to suggest a bronchial carcinoma.

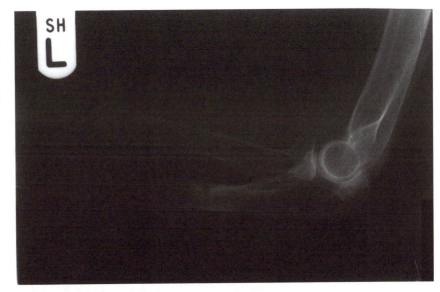

Case 28

This is a 95-year-old woman with pain in the forearm.

Question

28 What is the most likely diagnosis?
  ☐ A Fracture through a bony metastasis
  ☐ B Osteomalacia
  ☐ C Osteoporosis fracture from direct trauma.

Answer overleaf

Case 28

Answer

28   B   **Osteomalacia.**

Discussion

This forearm shows a generalised loss of bone density in the radius and ulna and in addition there is a lucency through the shaft of the ulna. The major radiological feature of osteomalacia is the presence of stress fractures or pseudofractures which are often referred to as Looser's zones.

There is a narrow radiolucent strip across the full thickness of the shaft of the ulna with slight sclerosis of the adjacent bone on either side.

This radiolucent strip may not extend across the full width of the bone particularly when these are seen in to upper femur. These are frequently bilateral and symmetrical and the common sites for these lesions are the pubic rami, scapulae, lower ribs, proximal femur and the ulna.

There is no major lytic process within the ulna which would be expected if this were a pathological fracture through a bony metastasis and bony metastases to the extremities are quite unusual except in bronchial carcinoma.

This would also be a very unusual site for a fracture due to direct trauma.

Case
28

**Case
29**

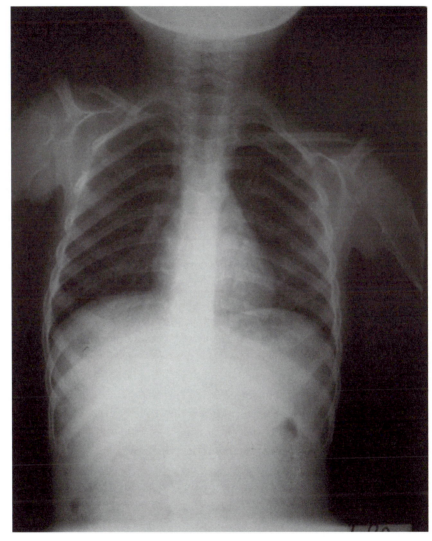

This is a 7-year-old boy with shoulder deformity.

Question

29   What is the most likely diagnosis?

☐   **A**   Achondroplasia

☐   **B**   Diaphyseal aclasis

☐   **C**   Cleidocranial dysostosis.

Answer overleaf

Case
29

Answer

29   B   **Diaphyseal aclasis.**

Discussion

This chest film shows a normal heart and normal mediastinum and lungs. There are, however, abnormalities of both upper humeri. There are multiple exostoses arising from the metaphyses of the humeri. These are multiple cartilage capped exostoses which are seen in diaphyseal aclasis. This is a hereditary condition in which multiple cartilage capped exostoses are present in the long bones.

Lesions may be present at birth but may not be noted until later childhood. The exostoses typically point away from the joint. There is a failure of bone modelling and the ends of the bones are often expanded. It chiefly affects the long bones with common sites being around the knee, the upper humerus, lower radius and ulna and both ends of the fibula. Malignant transformation occurs in about 5% of cases.

Achondroplasia typically affects short tubular bones which are relatively widened. The humerus and femur are most affected. The metaphyses are splayed with irregular ends and although the epiphyses are not affected they may be 'V' shaped.

In cranio cleido dysostosis the clavicles may be absent in part or altogether. This may be unilateral or bilateral. The outer end of the clavicle is more likely to be absent than the medial end.

Case 30

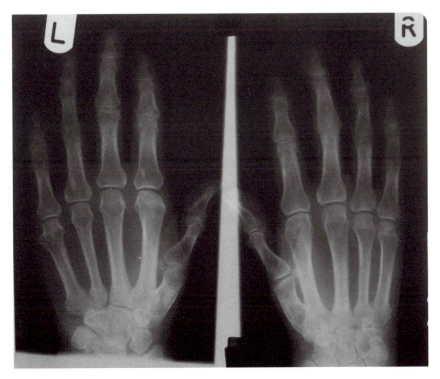

This is a 72-year-old man with stiff fingers.

Question

30   What is the most likely diagnosis?
   ☐   A   Rheumatoid arthritis
   ☐   B   Gout
   ☐   C   Old Still's disease
   ☐   D   Psoriatic arthropathy.

Answer overleaf

Answer

30   C   **Old Still's disease.**

Discussion

These hands show complete bony ankylosis across the proximal interphalangeal joints of the 3rd, 4th and 5th fingers. The joint spaces have become completely obliterated with the trabecular pattern of the bone continuing across the fused joints.

This is a late manifestation of juvenile chronic arthritis (Still's disease). In this condition although joint space narrowing and bone erosion are not as frequent as in rheumatoid arthritis, bony ankylosis of multiple joints may be the long term effect.

There are no erosions seen to indicate an active disease process. The first metacarpals are also somewhat short in this case.

In gout there may be soft tissue swelling around joints representing tophi which may be calcified and there are often juxta-atricular erosions.

In psoriatic arthropathy the distal interphalangeal joints are predominantly affected and there may be a relative lack of periarticular osteoporosis.

In rheumatoid arthritis the metacarpophalangeal joints are the common site of erosions and there is often marked periarticular osteoporosis and significant subluxation of joints and loss of joint space.

Case
31

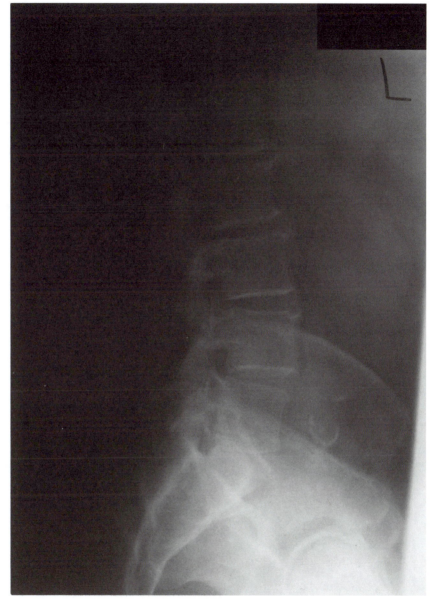

This is a 64-year-old man with a six-week history of back pain.

Question

31   What is the most likely diagnosis?

☐   **A**   Myeloma
☐   **B**   Infective discitis
☐   **C**   Abdominal aortic aneurysm
☐   **D**   Prolapsed intervertebral disc.

Answer overleaf

Case
31

Answer

31   C   **Abdominal aortic aneurysm**.

Discussion

This lateral lumbar spine view shows prominent anterior marginal osteophyte formation at several levels in the lumbar spine although the disc spaces are all well preserved. There is no evidence of any bony destruction. With a prolapsed intervertebral disc some loss of disc height would be expected.

With an infective discitis a narrowing of a disc space would be expected and some blurring of the vertebral end plates.

In myeloma some loss of bone density and loss of the trabecular pattern of the vertebral body, loss of height of the vertebral body and wedging might be evident. In addition the end plates might become indistinct.

The only abnormal feature here is the rim of calcification anterior to the lumbar spine which represents calcification in the wall of an aortic aneurysm.

A leaking aortic aneurysm may mimic pain from the lumbar spine. An abdominal CT scan of this patient confirmed the presence of an abdominal aortic aneurysm but did not show any evidence of a leak from the aneurysm.

Case
31

Case
32

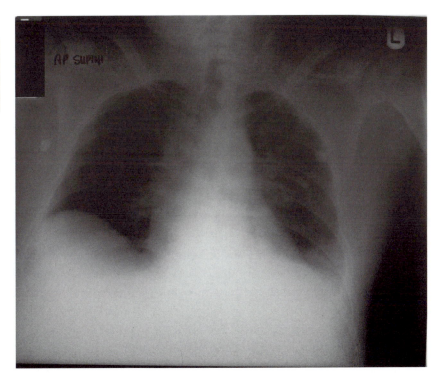

Film taken following insertion of central line.

Question

32   The tip of line is in either:

☐   A   The left main pulmonary artery

☐   B   Anomalous left pulmonary vein

☐   C   Coronary sinus

☐   D   Hemiazygous vein.

Answer overleaf

Case 32

Answer

32   B   **Anomalous left pulmonary vein.**

Discussion

Following an uncomplicated external jugular line insertion arterial blood was aspirated from the line. The chest radiograph showed that the tip of the central line was projected over the left lung.

A contrast study was carried out to further define where the catheter was sited (Figure 32A). This showed that the line had in fact entered an anomalous left pulmonary vein draining into the left innominate vein.

Anomalous pulmonary venous drainage is a spectrum ranging from total anomalous pulmonary venous drainage into the right atrium to minor abnormalities such as this. The most common anomalous pulmonary venous drainage is from the right upper lobe of the lung directly into the superior vena cava.

Left sided anomalous pulmonary venous drainage is rare but the majority of anomalous veins drain into the left innominate vein as in this case.

Other potential abnormal positions for external jugular catheters include the left hemiazygous vein which is a paravertebral vein draining into the left innominate vein or a persisting left superior vena cava draining into the coronary sinus.

This patient did not have a clinically significant left to right shunt.

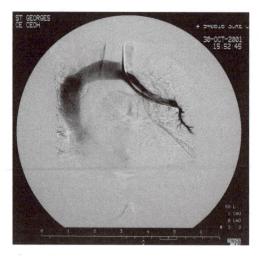

Figure 32A

Case
32

Case 33

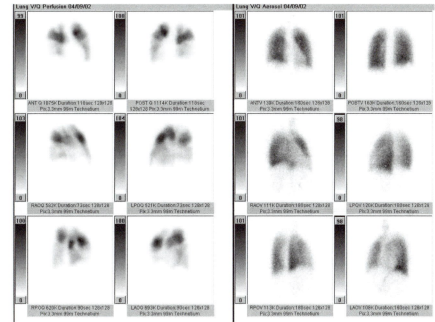

This 48-year-old man has a sudden onset of chest pain.

Question

33 What is the most likely diagnosis?

☐ **A** Right middle lobe collapse

☐ **B** Right middle lobe pneumonia

☐ **C** Pulmonary emboli

☐ **D** Pleural effusions.

Answer overleaf

Case 33

Answer

33   C   **Pulmonary emboli**.

Discussion

These are ventilation and perfusion lung scintigrams. The ventilation agent is ^{99m}Technetium labelled vaporised carbon particles. Alternatively ^{99m}Technetium aerosol or ^{81m}Krypton may be used.

There are multiple segmental defects on the perfusion images. These areas demonstrate normal ventilation. The findings on these images are therefore of multiple segmental areas of V/Q mismatch which carry a high probability for pulmonary embolism.

Collapse or atelectasis would give reduced perfusion and ventilation, described as matched defects. Pleural effusions also give matched defects, often at the bases if the effusion is uncomplicated.

In pneumonia there is reduced ventilation of the affected area, with slightly reduced or normal perfusion, described as reverse V/Q mismatch.

Case
33

Case 34

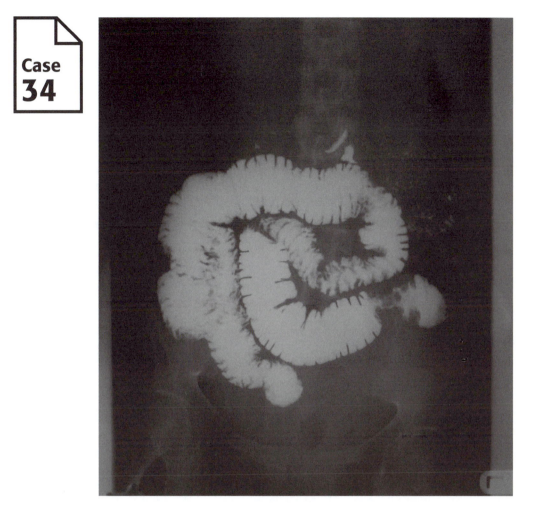

This is a 45-year-old patient with Coeliac disease.

Question

34   What is the most likely diagnosis?
  ☐   A   Chronic ulcerative jejunoileitis
  ☐   B   Amyloidosis
  ☐   C   Lymphoma
  ☐   D   Mesenteric lymphadenopathy.

Answer overleaf

Answer

34 C **Lymphoma**.

Discussion

This small bowel meal shows a narrowed segment of proximal small bowel with nodular filling defects within it extending over 2–3cm in length. The adjacent loops of small bowel are normal.

In uncomplicated coeliac disease the only abnormality seen on a small bowel study may be an increased separation of the mucosal folds in the proximal jejunum and an increase in the number of folds in the ileum.

Complications of coeliac disease include:
- hyposplenism
- enlarged mesenteric and retroperitoneal lymph nodes
- chronic ulcerative jejunoileitis
- enteropathy associated T-cell lymphoma
- carcinoma of the duodenum and upper jejunum.

Chronic ulcerative jejunoileitis is rare but is a serious complication and ulcers may bleed or the ulceration may lead to perforation. Subsequent stricture formation may produce small bowel obstruction. Chronic ulcerative jejunoileitis may be a precursor of lymphoma.

Enteropathy associated T-cell lymphoma is a serious complication of coeliac disease and once developed is highly malignant. On small bowel studies it can result in nodular fold thickening which may be discontinuous to more extensive mucosal ulceration and mass lesions such as seen here.

There is an increased incidence of carcinoma of the duodenum and jejunum in coeliac disease and in fact in this case the differential diagnosis of this lesion was either lymphoma or carcinoma. T-cell lymphoma was proven histologically.

Mesenteric lymphadenopathy may be seen in coeliac disease but in this case there is no evidence of separation of bowel loops which may be seen when there are enlarged mesenteric nodes.

Amyloid is not a recognised complication of coeliac disease and the radiological appearances are those of diffuse mucosal fold thickening.

See also Case 72.

Case 34

Case
35

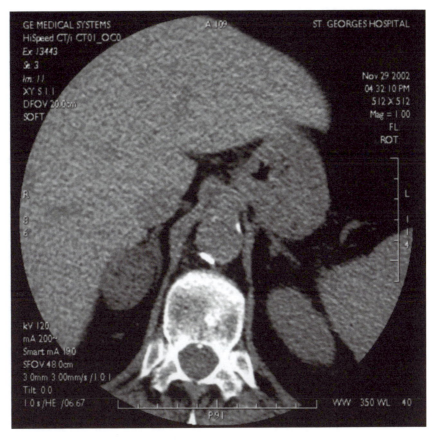

An incidental finding on CT of a 60-year-old woman.

Question

35   What is the most likely diagnosis?

    ☐   **A**   Adrenal tuberculosis

    ☐   **B**   Adrenal haemorrhage

    ☐   **C**   Neuroblastoma

    ☐   **D**   Adrenal adenoma.

Answer overleaf

Case
35

Answer

35   D   **Adrenal adenoma.**

Discussion

This is an unenhanced CT of the upper abdomen and shows a low density 2.5 cm diameter mass arising from the lateral limb of the right adrenal gland. It is of uniform density which is less than 10 Hounsfield units. The normal left adrenal gland is seen medial to the left crux of the diaphragm resembling an inverted 'V'.

Non-hyperfunctioning adrenal adenomas larger than 1 cm diameter can be seen incidentally in 1–3% of all upper abdominal CT examinations.

The number seen increases with age and they tend to occur in elderly women and in obese diabetics. These are typically of low density usually below 10 Hounsfield units. They have characteristics similar to functioning adrenal adenomas (Conn's tumour). They do not enhance significantly following iv contrast medium.

Adrenal haemorrhage is associated with severe trauma and of itself has no clinical signs. Non-traumatic haemorrhage is usually related to anticoagulation. Adrenal haemorrhage usually resolves but may result in calcification. An acute adrenal haemorrhage results in an adrenal gland of high attenuation.

Adrenal tuberculosis is usually bilateral and in active infection the glands are enlarged. During healing adrenal tuberculosis undergoes calcification and the glands may also atrophy.

Neuroblastoma is a tumour which is confined to children with a median age of presentation of 2 years.

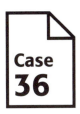

Case 36

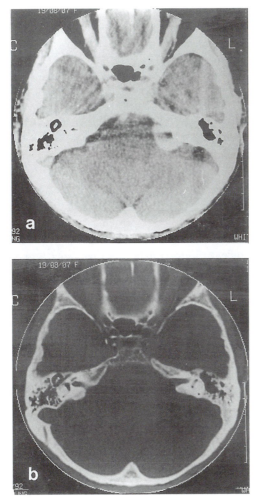

This 40-year-old patient presents with unilateral hearing loss.

Questions

36a   Describe *two* radiological abnormalities.

36b   What is the most likely diagnosis in this patient?
    ☐ A   Intracerebral haemorrhage
    ☐ B   Subdural haemorrhage
    ☐ C   Extradural haemorrhage
    ☐ D   Acoustic neuroma
    ☐ E   Meningioma
    ☐ F   Metastasis
    ☐ G   Glomus jugulare tumour.

Answer overleaf

Case 36

Answers

36a   The images are from a contrast-enhanced CT head scan of the posterior
        fossa on brain (a) and bone (b) settings.
   i There is a rounded, densely enhancing 2-cm mass in the left
      cerebellopontine angle. There is no associated calcification.
   ii There is widening of the left internal auditory canal (IAC) when
      compared with the right side.

36b   D   **A left-sided acoustic neuroma.**

Discussion

These are typical features of an acoustic neuroma which represent 80% of all
cerebellopontine angle tumours. Bilateral acoustic neuromas suggest
neurofibromatosis 2. Tumours less than 1 cm in size are not consistently
seen on CT, but essentially all are shown by contrast-enhanced MRI, the
radiological investigation of choice. Large tumours may cause
hydrocephalus.

Other causes of cerebellopontine angle masses include:
• Meningioma (10%): hyperdense mass pre-contrast, showing dense
  enhancement post-intravenous contrast. Unlike acoustic neuromas they
  are typically larger, may be calcified and tend to be broadly based along
  the petrous bone.
• Epidermoid (5%): low density mass on both pre- and post-contrast CT
  scans. This is the most common location for these fat-containing (hence
  low density) tumours.
• Others (5%): metastases (generally accompanied by bony erosion and a
  primary elsewhere), glomus jugulare tumour (associated erosion of the
  jugular foramen) and chordoma (most arise from the clivus).

The main differential diagnosis in this case is a meningioma, and widening
of the IAC is a useful discriminatory sign pointing to acoustic neuroma.

Case
36

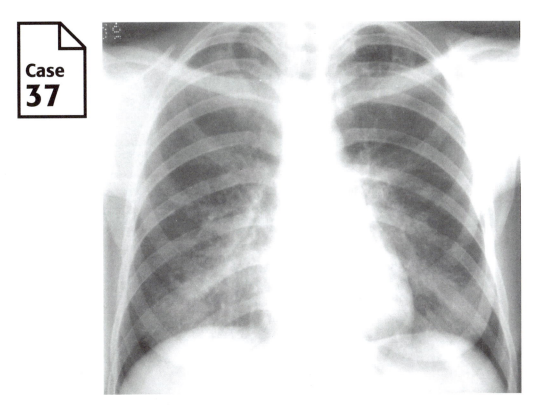

A 22-year-old patient with known malignancy undergoes chemotherapy. She becomes pyrexial and has a chest X-ray.

Question

37   What is the most likely diagnosis?

☐ A   Cardiac failure
☐ B   Lung abscess
☐ C   Opportunistic infection.

Answer overleaf

Case
37

Answer

37 C **Opportunistic infection**. The chest X-ray shows bilateral, perihilar air-space shadowing. The heart is of normal size and there are no pleural effusions, making cardiogenic oedema unlikely.

Discussion

The differential diagnosis includes:

- Opportunistic infection. Appearances are typical of *Pneumocystis carinii* pneumonia (the actual diagnosis) which is the commonest cause of opportunistic pulmonary infection in patients with the acquired immunodeficiency syndrome (AIDS). The chest radiograph is abnormal in 90% of cases, although it is often normal in the early stages. Common findings include a diffuse opacity of the lung parenchyma, which is often finely reticular in the early stages, but progresses to more confluent air-space shadowing with a tendency for perihilar accentuation. Pneumatoceles (arrow) – well defined air-spaces – may follow (Figure 37A). Pleural effusions and lymphadenopathy are rare. Cytomegalovirus infection causes a similar appearance. Seventy-five per cent of pulmonary complications in immunocompromised patients result from infection.
- Drug reaction.
- Pulmonary haemorrhage.
- Direct neoplastic involvement of the lung.

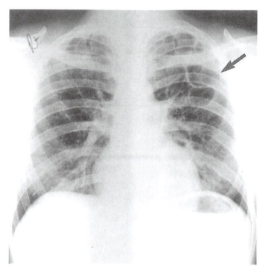

Figure 37A. Multiple pneumatoceles in both upper zones (arrow).

Case
37

Case 38

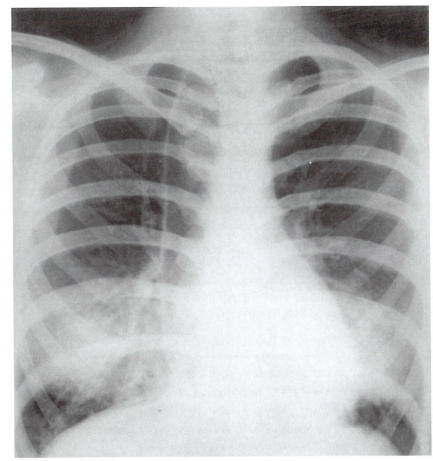

A 40-year-old woman presents with dysphagia.

Questions

38a   Describe *two* abnormalities on this chest radiograph.

38b   What is the most likely diagnosis?
- ☐   A   Pneumothorax
- ☐   B   Pleural effusion
- ☐   C   Carcinoma of the upper oesophagus
- ☐   D   Achalasia.

38c   What is the most likely complication that has occurred?
- ☐   A   Pneumothorax
- ☐   B   Pneumonia
- ☐   C   Lung metastases.

Answer overleaf   Case 38

Answers

38a   The chest X-ray demonstrates two abnormalities. There is an **abnormal linear opacity** extending from the diaphragm to the right of the superior mediastinum indicating a dilated oesophagus. In addition, there is **bilateral basal consolidation**.

38b   D   The primary abnormality in this patient is **achalasia**, but any obstruction to the distal oesophagus may cause this appearance.

38c   B   The most likely complication is **pneumonia** caused by aspiration of the oesophageal contents.

Discussion

Loss of propulsive peristaltic contractions, together with defective sphincter relaxation, results in a stasis of food and a progressively dilating and tortuous oesophagus. Additional radiographic features that may be seen include an air–fluid level visible in the mediastinum (or a mottled appearance due to a mixture of air and fluid). Generally little or no air is seen in the stomach.

Barium swallow classically shows a dilated oesophagus with smooth tapering of the lower end, likened to a rat's tail (Figure 38A).

Narrowing of the distal oesophagus is not specific to achalasia (although defective peristalsis and dilatation make this likely); it may also be seen in:
• Chagas' disease.
• Inflammatory strictures, e.g. due to reflux or corrosive ingestion.
• Neoplastic involvement: carcinoma of the oesophagus or stomach can cause an identical appearance either by direct involvement or by destruction of the myenteric plexus, although strictures are more commonly irregular.

Carcinoma is also a complication of longstanding achalasia.

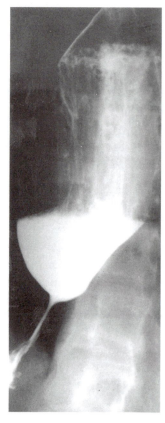

Figure 38A Achalasia on barium swallow.

Case **38**

Case
39

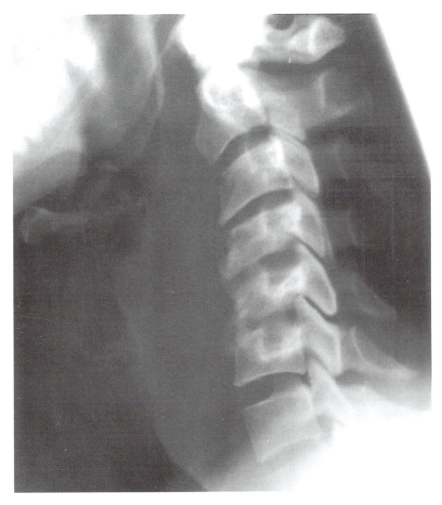

An Asian man presents with a painful neck.

Questions

39a   What *three* radiological abnormalities are seen in this X-ray?

39b   What is the most likely diagnosis?
- [ ] **A**   Bone metastases
- [ ] **B**   Degenerative disease
- [ ] **C**   Discitis
- [ ] **D**   Ankylosing spondylitis.

Answer overleaf

Case
39

Answers

39a   The lateral cervical spine X-ray demonstrates:
  i Narrowed disc-spaces at the C4/C5 and C5/C6 levels with loss of vertebral body height and destructive foci seen in the anterior corners of C3–C6.
  ii Marked precervical soft tissue swelling. Normally the precervical soft tissues measure <4 mm down to C4, beyond which they have the maximum width of a vertebral body.
  iii Reversal of the normal cervical lordosis.

39b C **Discitis.** In a patient of Asian origin, these appearances are most likely to be due to tuberculous spondylitis.

Discussion

Tuberculosis typically causes irregular bone destruction in a vertebral body, with narrowing of the adjacent intervertebral disc and extension of destruction across the disc to involve the contiguous vertebral body. Unlike pyogenic infection, tuberculous osteomyelitis is often associated with a paravertebral abscess and is rarely associated with bone sclerosis, but it is usually not possible to distinguish between the two on radiological criteria alone. Calcification when present indicates tuberculosis.

The lesions generally respond rapidly to anti-tuberculosis therapy and quiescence is evidenced by return of the bone detail and density and by the eroded bony margins becoming sharply defined.

Case
39

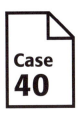

Case
40

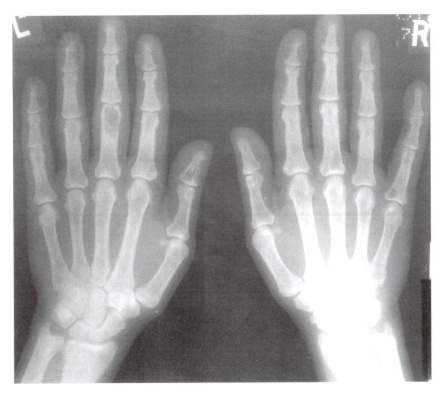

Questions

40a   What *three* radiological features are shown?

40b   What is the diagnosis?
- ☐ A   Bone metastases
- ☐ B   Rheumatoid arthritis
- ☐ C   Osteoarthritis
- ☐ D   Hyperparathyroidism
- ☐ E   Hypoparathyroidism.

Answer overleaf

Case
40

Answers

40a   i   Subperiosteal bone resorption, particularly affecting the radial side of the middle phalanx of the middle fingers. Other areas that may be involved include the lateral ends of the clavicles, medial aspect of the proximal tibia, pubic symphysis and the medial aspect of the neck of the femur.

      ii   Brown tumours: focal lytic lesions seen in the proximal phalanges of the left middle and right little fingers and also in the base of the terminal phalanx of the left thumb. These are locally destructive areas of intense osteoclastic activity and are most frequent in the mandible, ribs, pelvis and femora.

     iii   Resorption of the terminal tufts of the phalanges.

40b   D   **Hyperparathyroidism**
Radiological evidence of bone disease in hyperparathyroidism is no longer commonly seen (10% of cases).

Discussion

Additional radiological features that may be found include:
Bones:
- Osteopenia (uncommon).
- Diffuse cortical change – 'pepper-pot skull' (Figure 40A).
- Bone softening – basilar invagination, wedged or cod-fish vertebra.

Soft tissues:
- Soft tissue and periarticular calcifications.

Joints:
- Marginal erosions, but no joint space narrowing. Predominantly the distal interphalangeal joints.
- Chondrocalcinosis.

Kidney:
- Nephrocalcinosis.
- Calculi (in 50%).

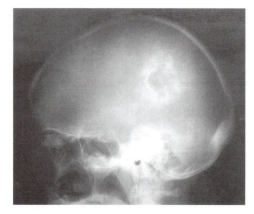

Figure 40A. 'Pepper-pot skull'.

Case
41

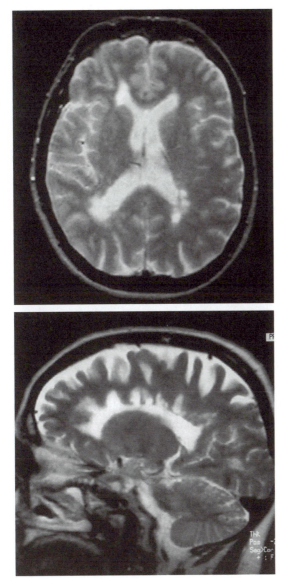

A 30-year-old woman undergoes an MRI scan.

Questions

41a   What does the T2-weighted MRI scan show?

41b   What is the most likely diagnosis?
   ☐ A   Syringomyelia
   ☐ B   Cerebellar hypoplasia
   ☐ C   Multiple sclerosis
   ☐ D   Glioblastoma
   ☐ E   Intraventricular haemorrhage.

Answer overleaf

Case
41

Answers

41a   Multiple, well-defined discrete foci of high signal intensity in the periventricular deep white matter of both hemispheres. The lesions are orientated perpendicular to the lateral ventricles and are not associated with mass effect.

41b   C   **Multiple sclerosis (MS)**
More than 85% of MS patients have ovoid periventricular lesions that are orientated perpendicularly to the long axis of the brain and lateral ventricles. The next most common site is the corpus callosum, involved in 50–90% of patients with clinically definite MS.

Discussion

In adults the brainstem and cerebellum are comparatively less common sites. Multiple lesions are typical and lesions may show enhancement with gadolinium on T1-weighted sequences up to 8 weeks following acute demyelination.

MS plaques (showing transient enhancement in the acute stage) may be seen on CT, but this is a less sensitive imaging modality than MRI.

Ischaemic lesions (areas of infarction) may have a similar appearance and patient age is useful in the distinction. In addition, the predominantly white-matter based lesions, particularly if they populate the roof of the lateral ventricles, favour the diagnosis of MS over infarction.

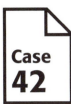

Case
42

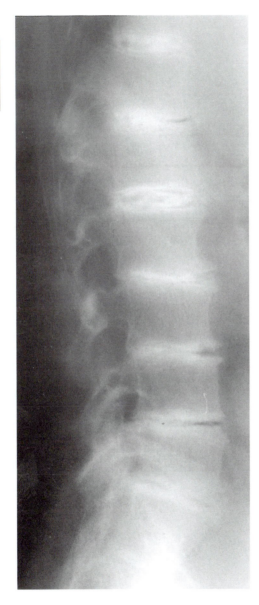

A 48-year-old man presents with a stiff back.

Question

42   What is the most likely diagnosis?
- ☐ **A**   Degenerative spondylosis
- ☐ **B**   Ankylosing spondylitis
- ☐ **C**   Juvenile rheumatoid arthritis
- ☐ **D**   Ochronosis.

Answer overleaf

Answer

42   D   **Ochronosis**.

Discussion

The lateral lumbar spine X-ray demonstrates dense laminated calcification of multiple invertebral discs. This is seen in the rare inborn error of metabolism, ochronosis, in which deposition of a pigment derivative of homogentisic acid is deposited in connective tissues producing a distinctive form of degenerative arthritis.

Intervertebral disc spaces are narrowed and limitation of movement is common. Severe, early degenerative arthritis may develop in peripheral joints, especially the shoulders, hips and knees. Chondrocalcinosis occurs and the sacroiliac joints may be affected.

Other causes of calcification of intervertebral discs include:
- Degenerative spondylosis: a frequent finding in the elderly.
- Transient calcification in children – commonly a self-limiting finding in the cervical spine.
- Calcium pyrophosphate dihydrate deposition disease. The deposits affect the annulus fibrosus and not the nucleus pulposus as in ochronosis.
- Ankylosing spondylitis – ankylosis, square vertebral bodies and syndesmophytes also seen.
- Less commonly – juvenile chronic arthritis, haemochromatosis, diffuse idiopathic skeletal hyperostosis, gout and post-traumatic.

Case
42

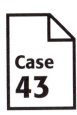

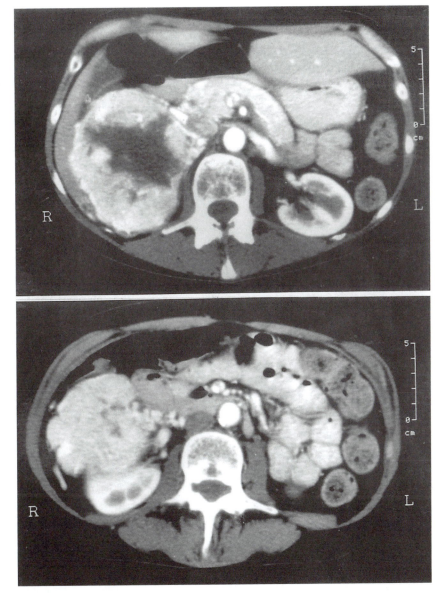

A 20-year-old girl presents with hypertension. The CT scans through the abdomen are post-intravenous contrast administration.

Question

43   What is the most likely diagnosis?

☐   A   Phaeochromocytoma

☐   B   Conn's tumour

☐   C   Renal cell-carcinoma

☐   D   Carcinoma of the head of the pancreas.

Answer overleaf   Case 43

Answer

43   A   The contrast-enhanced CT scans demonstrate a large (9 cm) well defined, rounded mass seen superior to the right kidney, which is inferiorly displaced. There is irregular rim enhancement with a central low attenuation region. The appearance is that of a right adrenal tumour with typical features of a **phaeochromocytoma**.

Discussion

The kidney is not involved, so renal cell-carcinoma is incorrect. Though the lesion is close to the head of the pancreas the epicentre of the lesion is the right adrenal gland. A Conn's adenoma is generally small homogeneous and of low density (due to cholesterol), making this diagnosis unlikely.

Phaeochromocytoma
At presentation these tumours are usually large (3–5 cm) and commonly show marked contrast enhancement, either rim or patchy.

The rule of 'tens' is useful:
• 10% are malignant, 10% bilateral, 10% extra-adrenal and 10% are multiple.
• 90% are sporadic, the remainder are inherited either as an isolated disorder or as part of a systemic disease, such as multiple endocrine neoplasia (MEN IIa or IIb), von Hippel–Lindau disease, or neurofibromatosis.

Other adrenal masses include:
Benign
• 'Non-functioning adenoma' ('incidentalomas'). Occur in 5%. Generally small and homogeneous.
• Cyst. Well-defined, water density.
• Angiomyolipoma. Usually 1–2 cm and contain areas of fat density.
• Haemorrhage. Hyperdense.
• Conn's adenoma. Generally small, homogeneous and of low density (due to cholesterol).
• Cushing's adenoma. Accounts for approximately 10% of Cushing's syndrome. Typically over 2 cm.
Malignant
Metastases. Usually larger than 2–3 cm, irregular with patchy enhancement. Can be bilateral.
Adrenal carcinoma. Generally larger than 6 cm, heterogenous with areas of necrosis and calcification. Can be functioning or non-functioning.
• Lymphoma. 25% also involve kidneys and lymphadenopathy is usually seen elsewhere.
• Neuroblastoma. Seen in infants. Calcification in 90%.

Case 43

Case 44

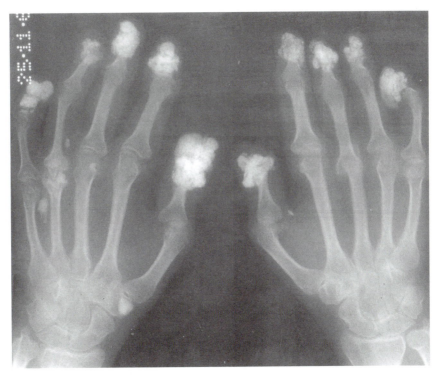

Question

44   What is the most likely diagnosis?

   ☐   A   Scleroderma

   ☐   B   Gout

   ☐   C   Tuberculosis

   ☐   D   Dermatomyositis

   ☐   E   Rheumatoid arthritis.

Answer overleaf

Case 44

Answer

44   A   The X-ray of the hands demonstrates: resorption of terminal phalangeal tufts; soft tissue calcifications, predominantly in the fingertips; generalized thinning of soft tissues with flexion contracture of the fingers (due to taut skin); reduced bone density (due to disease). The diagnosis is **scleroderma**.

Discussion

These changes are more common in the hands than in the feet. In 60% of cases there is resorption of distal phalangeal tufts. Calcific deposits are associated with soft tissue atrophy. Infrequently erosions similar to rheumatoid arthritis may develop (10%).

Gastrointestinal involvement occurs in 50% (most commonly atonic dilated oesophagus), interstitial fibrotic lung disease in 25% and cardiac involvement with cardiomyopathy in 35%.

Other causes of soft tissue calcification:
- Dermatomyositis – extensive calcifications may be seen in muscles and subcutaneous tissues underlying the skin lesions, as shown in Figure 44A.
- Metabolic: Calcified tophi are seen in gout but these are associated with the joints (the first metatarsal phalangeal joint is most commonly affected). Hyperparathyroidism may cause soft tissue calcification, more commonly in the secondary form, and vascular calcification is often seen.
- Infective tuberculous nodes may cause soft tissue calcification but the site and distribution would be at the lymph node groups.
- Traumatic: calcified haematoma.
- Myositis ossificans (outer part is more densely calcified than the centre).
- Parasitic calcification, e.g. *Loa loa*, cysticercosis.
- Rheumatoid arthritis does not cause calcification.

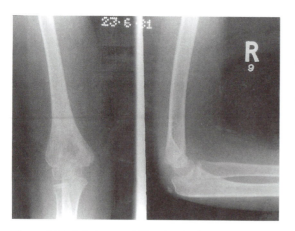

Figure 44A Soft tissue calcification in dermatomyositis.

Case
44

Case **45**

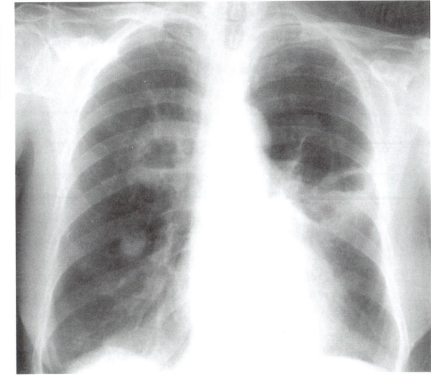

Question

45   Which of the following diagnoses would *not* cause this chest X-ray appearance?

    ☐   A   Infection

    ☐   B   Wegener's granulomatosis

    ☐   C   Hodgkin's disease

    ☐   D   Rheumatoid arthritis

    ☐   E   Trauma

    ☐   F   Bullous emphysema.

Answer overleaf   Case **45**

Answer

45   F   **Bullous emphysema**.

Discussion

In bullous emphysema large bullae occur which are radiolucent and thin walled. The chest X-ray in this question, however, shows thick-walled cavitating lesions and other soft tissue pulmonary masses.

There are many causes of multiple cavitating lung masses:
- Infective: likely pathogens include *Staphylococcus aureus* (particularly in children), *Klebsiella pneumoniae* and tuberculosis.

Neoplastic:
- Metastases – seen especially in squamous cell tumours (two-thirds).
- Hodgkin's disease – hilar or medistinal lymphadenopathy generally also present.
- Vascular: Infarction – either due to septic emboli or infection of initially sterile infarcts.
- Granulomas: Wegener's involved and cavitation is common (30–50%). Lesions are typically thick-walled. Nodules may be partially or completely resolved and do not calcify.
- Rheumatoid nodules – also thick-walled, especially in the lower lobes. Tend to be peripheral and well-defined.
- Sarcoidosis (rare presentation).
- Traumatic: Haematoma – usually subpleural and under point of maximal injury. Resolves slowly. Rib fractures are also often seen.

A useful mnemonic is *CAVIT*: *C*arcinoma, *A*utoimmune disease, *V*ascular, *I*nfection, *T*rauma. Ultimately clinical details are necessary to help differentiate between the numerous causes.

Case 46

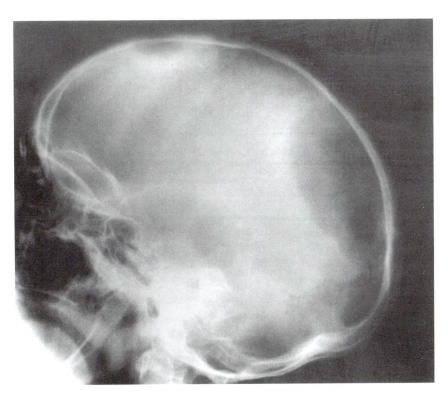

A 70-year-old man has a skull X-ray.

Question

46   What is the most appropriate diagnosis?
  ☐ **A**   Paget's disease
  ☐ **B**   Carcinoma of the prostate
  ☐ **C**   Acromegaly
  ☐ **D**   Multiple myeloma.

Answer overleaf   Case 46

Answer

46   A   **Paget's disease.**

Discussion

The lateral skull X-ray demonstrates a large, sharply defined lytic lesion involving the parietal and occipital regions and a similar smaller lytic lesion in the frontal bone – osteoporosis circumscripta.

Basiliar invagination is another abnormality shown. The tip of the odontoid peg is normally less than 0.5 cm above McGregor's line (connecting the occiput to the posterior end of the hard palate).

Osteoporosis circumscripta occurs in the active lytic phase of the disease and starts in the lower parts of the frontal and occipital regions and can cross suture lines to involve large areas of the skull vault. Later, in the sclerotic phase, the skull vault thickens and 'cotton wool' sclerotic areas of bone are seen (Figure 46A). The facial bones are not commonly affected. Paget's disease affects 10% of the population in old age.

Other causes of lucencies in the skull vault of an *adult* are:
- Multiple myeloma: lesions have a 'punched out' appearance and can affect the mandible, which metastases rarely do.
- Metastases: generally ill-defined and irregular. Common primary tumours are breast, kidney and thyroid.
- Burr hole: well-defined. History of previous surgery.
- Hyperparathyroidism: 'pepper-pot' skull – which is not often severe enough to cause distinct lytic lesions. Basilar invagination may occur and brown tumours may be seen.
- Infective: (including tuberculosis).
- Rarely: haemangioma and neurofibroma.

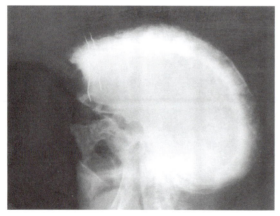

Figure 46A The skull is affected in 65% of cases of Paget's disease. The hair clip is an artefact.

Case
46

Case 47

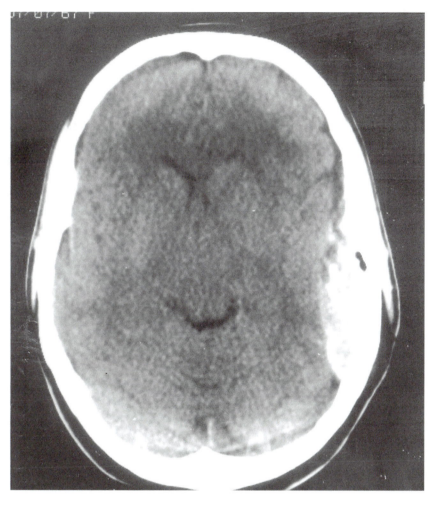

A 30-year-old man involved in a road traffic accident. He has an unenhanced CT scan of his brain.

Question

47   What is the most likely diagnosis?
- ☐ A   Subarachnoid haemorrhage
- ☐ B   Subdural haemorrhage
- ☐ C   Extradural haematoma
- ☐ D   Intracerebral haemorrhage.

Answer overleaf

Case 47

Answer

47   C   **Extradural haematoma**.

Discussion

The unenhanced CT scan of the head demonstrates a moderate sized, high attenuation, lenticular shaped left extradural haematoma in the temporoparietal region. The heterogenous density of the collection is suggestive of active bleeding.

Intracranial air (pneumocephalus) – an air loculus is seen adjacent to the extradural haematoma. It is indicative of a base of skull fracture, or fracture through the paranasal air sinuses.

There is mass effect and shift of the midline structures from left to right.

Extradural haematoma occurs in a temporoparietal location in 66% of cases and is associated with a skull fracture in 40–85%. Note the biconvex shape compared with the crescenteric shape of a subdural haematoma. Extradural haematomas are dangerous because of focal mass effect and rapid onset.

Intracranial haemorrhage means that there is bleeding within the head. It is further subdivided into extradural which means bleeding has occurred between the skull and the dura, subdural which means bleeding has occurred between the dura and the pia (the delicate membrane covering the brain); subarachnoid which means bleeding has occurred into the CSF spaces and intracerebral which means bleeding has occurred within the brain parenchyma.

Case
47

Case
48

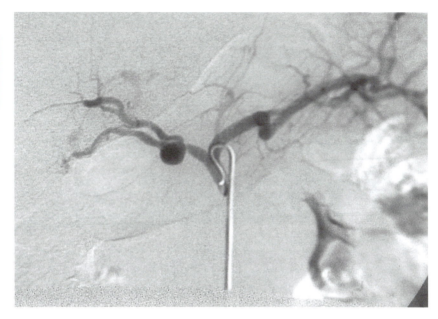

A 30-year-old female has a history of weight loss, hypertension and an elevated ESR. A coeliac axis angiogram is shown.

Question

48   What is the most likely diagnosis?
- ☐ A   Carcinoma of the head of the pancreas
- ☐ B   Polyarteritis nodosa
- ☐ C   Acute gastrointestinal bleed
- ☐ D   Arteriovenous malformation.

Answer overleaf

Case
48

Answer

48   B   **Polyarteritis nodosa**.

Discussion

The coeliac axis angiogram demonstrates a solitary saccular hepatic artery aneurysm arising from a common hepatic artery prior to its bifurcation.

Polyarteritis nodosa is a systemic connective tissue disorder characterised by focal areas of necrotizing arteritis with aneurysm formation.

All organs may be involved: kidney (85%), heart (65%), liver (50%), pancreas, bowel, CNS (cerebrovascular accident, seizure).

Hepatic or renal angiograms show characteristic 1–5 mm saccular aneurysms, typically involving small to medium sized arteries (60–75%) and commonly multiple. The kidney may be normal in size, enlarged, shrunken from glomerulonephritis or scarred from infarction.

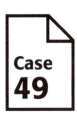

Case 49

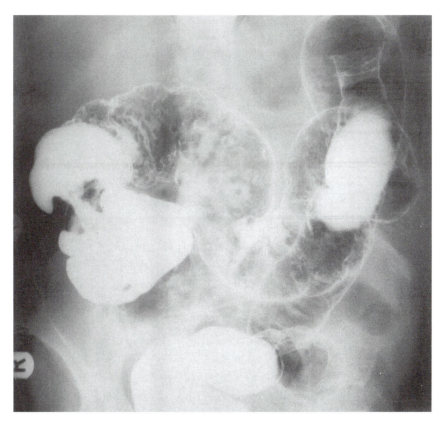

A 30-year-old man presents with abdominal pain and weight loss. His barium enema is shown.

Question

49   Choose *two* diagnoses which accounts for the appearance.

☐   A   Carcinoma of the sigmoid colon
☐   B   Carcinoma of the ascending colon
☐   C   Polyposis coli syndrome
☐   D   Crohn's disease
☐   E   Ulcerative colitis
☐   F   Diverticular disease
☐   G   Pneumatosis coli.

Answer overleaf   Case 49

Answer

49   B, C   **Polyposis coli syndrome** with an associated **carcinoma** of the ascending colon.

Discussion

The barium enema demonstrates:
- Multiple round filling defects throughout the colon consistent with sessile polyps of varying size.
- A large annular carcinoma of the ascending colon.

Multiple intestinal polyps occur in a number of syndromes and clinical information is needed to help differentiate:
- Familial polyposis coli – autosomal dominant. Multiple adenomatous polyps (usually about 1000) appear around puberty. 2–3 mm polyps (up to 2 cm) are usually scattered evenly from rectum to caecum. Malignant transformation occurs in 100% by 20 years after diagnosis. Treatment is prophylactic total colectomy. Associated with hamartomas of stomach (49%), adenomas of duodenum (25%) and periampullary carcinoma.
- Gardner's syndrome – autosomal dominant. Characterised by colonic adenomatous polyposis (indistinguishable from familial polyposis coli). Multiple osteomata of the mandible and skull and soft tissue tumours occur. Eventual malignant transformation of polyps in 100%. Associated with periampullary carcinoma, thyroid and adrenal carcinoma.
- Peutz–Jegher's syndrome – autosomal dominant. Characterised by benign

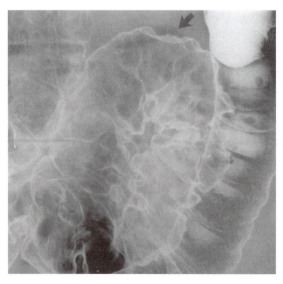

hamartomatous intestinal polyposis and mucocutaneous pigmentation. Polyps most numerous in small bowel (>95%) compared with the colon (30%). Complications include intussusception.

Differentiation from pneumatosis coli (Figure 49A) is usually easy since the air cysts extend outside the mucosal line (arrow).

Figure 49A Pneumatosis coli. The left half of the colon is the site most commonly affected.

Case
49

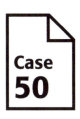

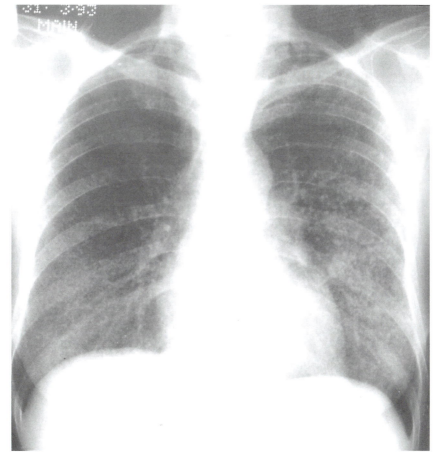

An 18-year-old patient from abroad who is unwell.

Question

50 What is the most likely diagnosis?
- ☐ A Miliary tuberculosis
- ☐ B Miliary metastases
- ☐ C Cardiac failure
- ☐ D Pericardial effusion.

Answer overleaf

Answer

50   A   **Miliary tuberculosis.**

Discussion

The chest X-ray demonstrates widespread bilateral miliary nodular shadowing. There is no associated hilar or mediastinal lymphadenopathy.

In an ill patient, miliary tuberculosis is the most likely diagnosis and the *pre-eminent* consideration as prompt diagnosis and treatment are vital.

Miliary tuberculosis (TB), which results from haematogenous dissemination of the disease, is an infrequent but feared complication of both primary and reactivation TB. Radiographically, the result is widespread small (1 mm) nodules, which are uniformly distributed and equal in size (likened in size and appearance to millet seeds). Hila are normal unless superimposed on primary TB. As there is a threshold below which the nodules are invisible, miliary TB can be present in a patient whose chest radiograph appears normal. Even with successful treatment, the miliary nodulation may take weeks or months to clear.

Other causes of miliary shadowing to consider are:
• Metastases: most commonly from papillary or follicular thyroid carcinoma.
• Coal miner's pneumoconiosis – predominantly in mid-zones.
• Fungal diseases, e.g. histoplasmosis, coccidioidomycosis.
• Sarcoidosis: predominantly mid-zones, often with enlarged hilar.
• Acute extrinsic allergic alveolitis – initially most prominent in the lower zones. Poorly defined.

Case 51

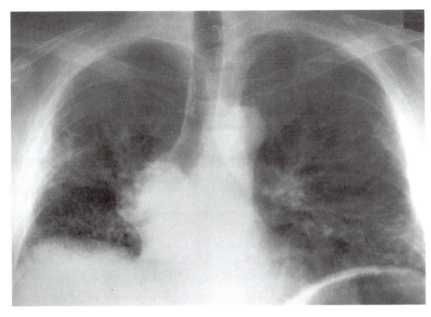

A 50-year-old male with dyspnoea and finger clubbing.

Question

51   What are the *two* most likely diagnoses?

☐   A   Bronchial carcinoma
☐   B   Lung abscess
☐   C   Dextrocardia
☐   D   Cryptogenic fibrosing alveolitis
☐   E   Sarcoidosis.

Answer overleaf

Case 51

Answer

51   A, D   **Bronchial carcinoma** and **cryptogenic fibrosing alveolitis (CFA)**.

Discussion

The chest X-ray demonstrates: (i) bilateral mid and lower zone reticular shadowing with obscuration of pulmonary vascular markings and loss of a sharp cardiac outline; (ii) reduced lung volumes; (iii) large, soft tissue density mass projected over the right hilum.

Certain radiographic features help distinguish between the many causes of pulmonary fibrosis:
- Distribution: those conditions showing basal predominance include CFA, drug-related fibrosis, connective tissue disorders (scleroderma, rheumatoid arthritis) and asbestosis. Mid and upper zone predominance favours sarcoidosis, previous tuberculosis, ankylosing spondylitis, chronic extrinsic allergic alveolitis.
- Pleural disease: calcified pleural plaques suggest previous asbestos exposure. Pleural effusions are rare in CFA, sarcoidosis and scleroderma and suggest connective tissue disorders.
- Lymphadenopathy: 75–85% of patients with sarcoidosis have nodal enlargement at some time.

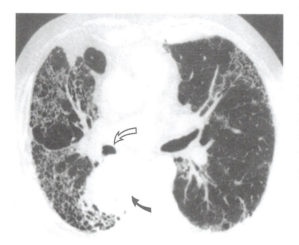

Additionally, erosion of the ends of the clavicles may be seen in rheumatoid arthritis and a dilated oesophagus (± air fluid level) is most suggestive of scleroderma.

In this case, in the absence of previous drug therapy, the most likely diagnosis is CFA, particularly in view of finger clubbing. Carcinoma of the lung is 14 times more common in people with CFA than in the general population.

Figure 51A Thin section CT scan demonstrating a characteristic coarse, subpleural reticular pattern compatible with an established fibrosing alveolitis. The bronchogenic carcinoma (arrow) is seen posterior to the right main bronchus (open arrow).

Case
51

Case 52

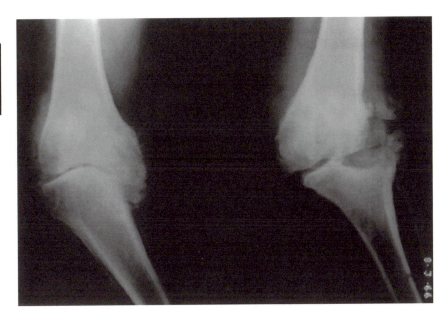

X-ray of both knees.

Question

52   What is the most likely diagnosis?
- ☐ A   Neuropathic (Charcot's) joints
- ☐ B   Rheumatoid arthritis
- ☐ C   Osteoarthritis
- ☐ D   Osteomalacia
- ☐ E   Osteoporosis
- ☐ F   Metastatic disease.

Answer overleaf

Case 52

Answer

52   A   **Neuropathic (Charcot's) joints**.

Discussion

The X-rays demonstrate severe bilateral knee joint destruction, subluxation and heterotopic new bone (debris). The most likely diagnosis is neuropathic (Charcot's) joints.

A neuropathic joint is severely destroyed and disorganised. The process is painless, allowing the patient to continue to weight bear, which can cause further damage to the joint.

The most common cause of a Charcot joint is in the foot of a diabetic (typically the first and second tarsometatarsal joints). Other causes include tabes dorsalis and syphilis which predominantly affect the weight-bearing joints of the lower extremities and lower lumbar spine. Other causes include syringomyelia (the shoulder can become a Charcot joint). Neuropathic joints may also occur in congenital indifference to pain, leprosy, spinal cord injury, spina bifida and alcoholism.

Other processes such as tuberculosis may completely destroy a joint but the process is painful and although a radiograph may look similar, the term Charcot joint cannot be applied as this is strictly reserved for neuropathic joints, that is where a damaged nerve supply is the primary cause.

Case
52

Case 53

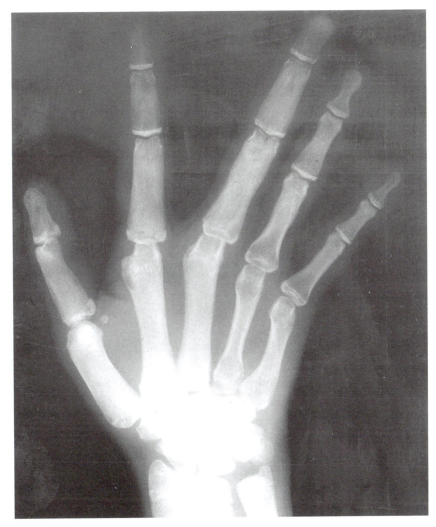

Hand X-ray of a 10-year-old girl with precocious puberty.

Question

53   What is the most likely diagnosis?

- ☐ A   Paget's disease
- ☐ B   McCune–Albright syndrome
- ☐ C   Turner's syndrome
- ☐ D   Acromegaly.

Answer overleaf   **Case 53**

Answer

53   B   **McCune–Albright syndrome**.

Discussion

Turner's syndrome does not cause precocious puberty. In the hand it may produce a false metacarpal. Note, however, that the fourth and fifth fingers are normal in this case but the expansion and modelling deformity affects the thumb, index and middle fingers, making the digits of the fourth and fifth fingers look small.

McCune–Albright syndrome (MAS) is characterised by the clinical triad of polyostotic fibrous dysplasia, café-au-lait skin pigmentation and multiple endocrinopathies. Precocious puberty is the commonest initial presentation, but other endocrinopathies that have been described include hyperthyroidism, growth hormone excess, hyperprolactinaemia, Cushing's syndrome and hypophosphataemic osteomalacia. MAS is not inherited, but occurs as a sporadic condition.

Polyostotic fibrous dysplasia typically develops before the age of 10 years, presenting with pain, swelling, fracture or deformity. The normal bone is replaced by fibrous vascular tissue. Skull involvement may result in severe deformities, unilateral exophthalmos and cranial nerve symptoms due to foraminal obliteration.

Malignant degeneration is rare.

Paget's disease may show similar features but affects older patients (typically over 60 years).

Case
53

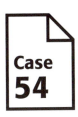

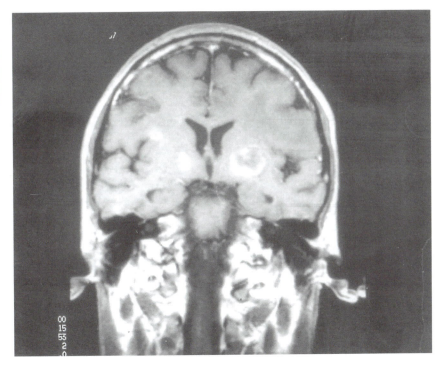

This is a coronal, T1-weighted, contrast-enhanced MRI scan, in a 26-year-old male with AIDS.

Question

54   What is the most likely diagnosis?
- [ ] A   Toxoplasmosis
- [ ] B   Lymphoma
- [ ] C   Multiple metastasis
- [ ] D   Intracerebral abscesses
- [ ] E   Cytomegalovirus infection.

Answer overleaf

Answer

54   A   **Toxoplasmosis.**

Discussion

The T1-weighted contrast-enhanced MRI scan of the brain of a 26-year-old male with AIDS demonstrates multiple lesions in both cerebral hemispheres which typically show ring enhancement. Lesions are seen in both basal ganglia.

Toxoplasmosis is caused by the intracellular parasite *Toxoplasma gondii* and it is the most common opportunistic CNS infection in patients with AIDS. The basal ganglia and cerebral hemispheres near the cortico-medullary junction are the most common sites.

Contrast-enhanced CT scans show solitary (up to 40%) or multiple ring-enhancing masses with peripheral oedema.

Lesions are typically iso- to slightly hypointense on T1-weighted MRI scans. Focal nodular or rim enhancement patterns are seen following contrast administration. Treated lesions often demonstrate calcification or haemorrhage.

The major differential diagnostic consideration is primary CNS lymphoma (Figure 54A). The detection of more than one lesion favours toxoplasmosis; periventricular location and subependymal spread favour lymphoma.

CNS lymphoma affects 6% of AIDS patients. 50% display uniform contrast enhancement and 50% show ring enhancement. Solitary lesions are present in 50% of cases and are often associated with oedema (as in Figure 54A).

Multiple abscesses and metastases may cause ring-enhancing lesions but given the clinical context toxoplasmosis is most likely. Cytomegalovirus tends to cause a retinitis.

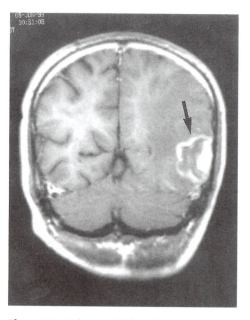

Figure 54A Primary CNS lymphoma (arrow) on a coronal T1-weighted MRI brain scan.

Case
54

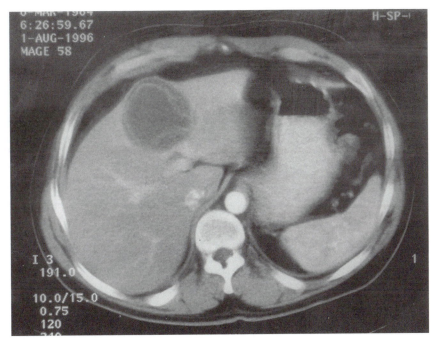

Contrast-enhanced CT scan through the upper abdomen.

Question

55   What is the most likely diagnosis?
   - ☐ A   Amoebic abscess
   - ☐ B   Metastasis
   - ☐ C   Hydatid cyst
   - ☐ D   Acute cholecystitis
   - ☐ E   Empyema.

Answer overleaf

Answer

55   C   **Hydatid (echinococcal) cyst.**

Discussion

There is a large non-calcified, low attenuation, thin-walled, cystic lesion within the liver. It is unilocular but a thin, wavy membrane is seen inside the cyst towards the periphery. The gallbladder is not seen and would be at a lower level in the abdomen.

Tissue infection of humans is caused by the larval stage of a small tapeworm for which dogs, sheep, cattle and camels are the major intermediate hosts.

A large single hepatic cyst or multiple well-defined cystic lesions may be seen and are often asymptomatic for many years. On CT scan they are rounded, near-water attenuation masses with thin walls. They may appear multilocular with internal septations representing thin walls of daughter cysts. Cyst walls may show dense calcification and gas may occur within (due to superimposed infection or communication with the biliary tree). When detached from the pericyst the true cyst wall may appear as a thin wavy membrane (as above).

Other causes of cystic lesions within the liver are:
- Simple, congenital cyst: (common). Single or multiple. No internal septations. Smooth walls.
- Polycystic disease: multiple low attenuation cysts of various sizes, associated with polycystic kidneys.
  Abscesses: including pyogenic and amoebic. May also contain gas.
- Metastases: cystic metastases (sarcoma, melanoma, ovarian and colon carcinoma) may closely simulate benign cysts, though they often have shaggy and irregular walls (Figure 55A).

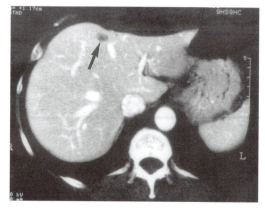

Figure 55A CT scan of the liver. Solitary, irregular metastasis from colonic carcinoma (arrow). Cystic nature confirmed on ultrasound.

Case
55

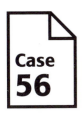

Case 56

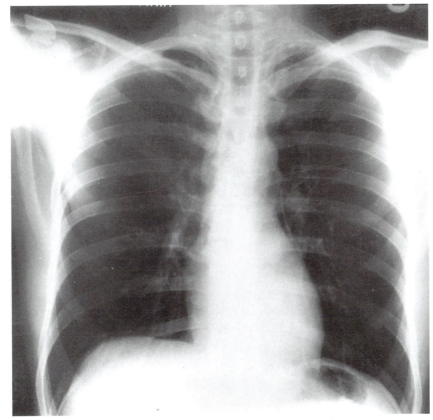

A 25-year-old presenting with chest pain following an episode of food poisoning.

Question

56   What is the most likely diagnosis?
- ☐ A   Pneumothorax
- ☐ B   Oesophageal rupture
- ☐ C   Aortic dissection
- ☐ D   Pericarditis
- ☐ E   Endocarditis.

Answer overleaf   Case **56**

Answer

56 B **Oesophageal rupture (Boerhaave's syndrome)**, due to excessive vomiting.

Discussion

The chest X-ray demonstrates a pneumomediastinum. Vertical streaks of air in the mediastinum are best seen in the region of the left hilum where the pleura is visualised as a linear opacity parallel to the mediastinum. The pleura is not normally visible as a line but is seen here because there is air on both sides of it, i.e. air within the lung which is *normal* and air within the mediastinum which is *abnormal*. The air is usually greatest in amount anteriorly and this is often more obvious on the lateral view. Surgical emphysema and pneumothorax may be associated features.

Causes of a pneumomediastinum can be divided into:
- Alveolar rupture:
  Spontaneous – generally in healthy young patients following a bout of coughing or vomiting.
  Mechanical ventilation.
  Following compressive thoracic trauma.
  Following rupture of a lung by rib fracture.
- Traumatic laceration of the trachea or a central bronchus.
- Perforation of the oesophagus:
  Spontaneous.
  Following instrumentation.
- Perforation of pharynx, duodenum, colon or rectum with tracking of air into the mediastinum.

Symptoms include chest pain and dyspnoea. Fever and leucocytosis are frequently seen.

Case
56

Case 57

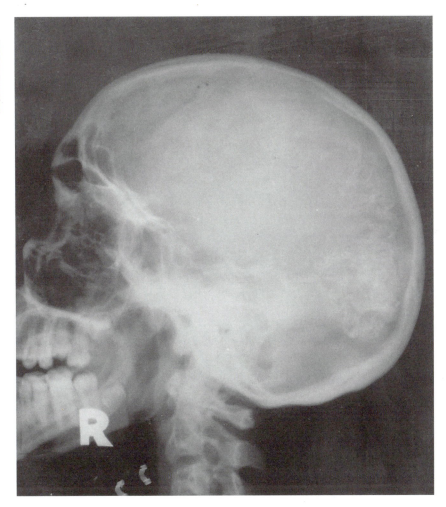

This young man presents with epilepsy.

Question

57   What is the diagnosis?

☐ A   Acromegaly
☐ B   Calcification of the choroid plexus
☐ C   Sturge–Weber syndrome
☐ D   Paget's disease.

Answer overleaf

Case 57

Answer

57   C   **Sturge–Weber syndrome.**

Discussion

The lateral skull X-ray demonstrates characteristic tram-track, gyriform plaques of calcification. The calcification is in the brain cortex and follows the cerebral convolutions, most often displaying in the parieto-occipital area.

It is due to a congenital vascular anomaly in which a localised meningeal venous angioma occurs in conjunction with an ipsilateral facial angioma (port wine naevus). The clinical findings include mental retardation (>50%), seizures (90%), hemiatrophy and hemiparesis.

Additional radiological abnormalities, better demonstrated on CT scan include: cortical hemiatrophy, ipsilateral thickening of the skull and enlargement of ipsilateral paranasal air sinuses.

Intracranial calcifications may also be due to:
- Physiological causes, e.g. choroid plexus/pineal calcification. Calcification is physiological and it does not result in epilepsy.
- Infection: toxoplasmosis, rubella, cytomegalovirus, *Herpes simplex,* cysticercosis, tuberculosis.
- Neoplasm: craniopharyngioma (40–80%), oligodendroglioma (50–70%), chordoma (25–40%), meningioma (20%).
- Endocrine: hyperparathyroidism, hypoparathyroidism.
- Toxic: carbon monoxide, lead poisoning.
- Embryologic: tuberous sclerosis, neurofibromatosis.
- Vascular: aneurysm, arteriovenous malformation, subdural haematoma.

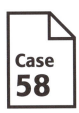

Case 58

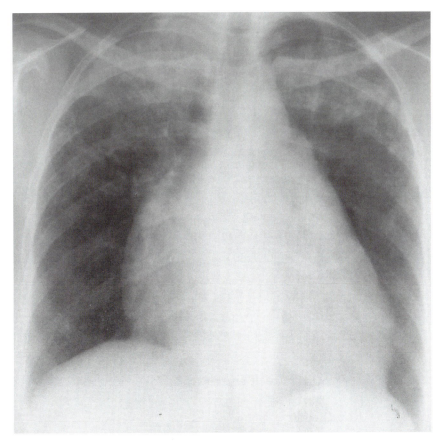

A 25-year-old male with a fever. The chest X-ray taken one week previously was normal.

Question

58 What is the diagnosis?
- ☐ A   Cardiac failure
- ☐ B   Sarcoid
- ☐ C   Tuberculosis
- ☐ D   Myocardial infarction.

Answer overleaf

Answer

58   C   The cardiac silhouette is suggestive of a pericardial effusion. There is also bilateral upper lobe air space shadowing. In the presence of a fever the findings should suggest the possibility of **tuberculosis** – especially in an Asian patient.

Discussion

Other causes of gross cardiomegaly are:
• Multiple valvular disease – aortic and mitral valve disease, particularly with regurgitation.
• Cardiomyopathy (including ischaemic).
• Atrial septal defect.

Plain film appearances of a pericardial effusion depend on the amount of pericardial fluid present. The cardiac silhouette may be globular or have a non-specific shape, but with no specific features to suggest selective chamber enlargement (as will be the case in some of the other causes listed).

Causes of a pericardial effusion include:
• Infective (bacterial, tuberculous or viral)
• Malignancy
• Dressler's syndrome
• Myxoedema
• Systemic lupus erythematosus
• Uraemia
• Trauma.

Case
58

Case
59

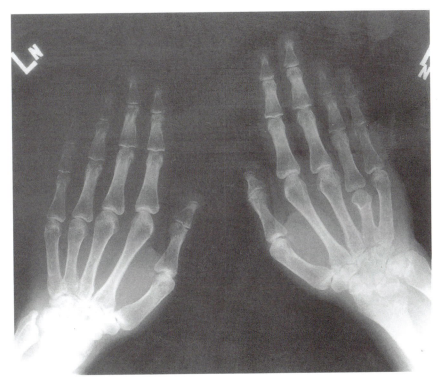

Question

59   What is the most likely diagnosis?

☐   A   Hyperparathyroidism

☐   B   Hypoparathyroidism

☐   C   Pseudohypoparathyroidism

☐   D   Acromegaly.

Answer overleaf   Case **59**

Answer

59   C   **Pseudohypoparathyroidism**.

Discussion

There is shortening of the right and (to a lesser extent) the left fourth metacarpal. A tangent between the third and fifth metacarpals normally intersects the fourth.

Other causes of this appearance include pseudopseudohypopara-thyroidism and Turner's syndrome.

The principal radiological findings in pseudohypoparathyroidism are short stature with short metacarpals, metatarsals and phalanges, particularly the fourth and fifth metacarpals. Calcification may be present in the basal ganglia, cerebellum and skin.

Pseudopseudohypoparathyroidism presents the same skeletal syndrome, but with normal blood chemistry.

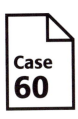

Case
60

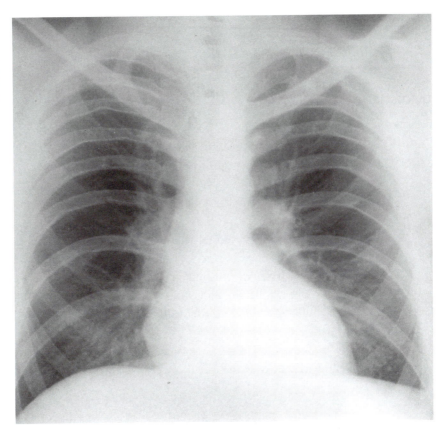

A 26-year-old man is found to be hypertensive at an insurance medical examination.

Question

60   What is the most likely diagnosis?
- ☐ A   Atrial septal defect
- ☐ B   Ventricular septal defect
- ☐ C   Coarctation of the aorta
- ☐ D   Vasculitus
- ☐ E   Fallot's tetralogy.

Answer overleaf

Case
60

Answer

60   C   **Coarctation of the aorta**.

Discussion

There is notching of the inferior aspects of the posterior ribs bilaterally, sparing the upper two ribs. The heart is not enlarged but the aortic knuckle has an abnormal 'figure 3' configuration.

Coarctation of the aorta refers to an area of localised narrowing. It is most commonly congenital and may be either preductal or postductal in location.

The chest radiograph shows rib notching (caused by dilatation and tortuosity of the intercostal arteries) affecting the inferior surfaces of the posterior rib elements, but not usually seen before the second decade. Generally rib notching is bilateral and spares the first two ribs.

The aortic knuckle can have an abnormal 'figure 3' configuration caused by the dilated origin of the left subclavian artery and poststenotic dilatation of the arch.

Cardiomegaly suggests associated aortic valve disease, and signs of cardiac failure may be present.

Other causes of inferior rib notching include:
• Neurofibromatosis – 'ribbon ribs' may also be a feature.
• Superior vena cava obstruction.
• Pulmonary oligaemia – any cause of decreased pulmonary blood supply.
• Subclavian obstruction – most commonly post-Blalock operation for Fallot's tetralogy, which typically leads to unilateral rib notching of the upper three or four ribs on the operation side.

Associations of coarctation of the aorta include Turner's syndrome (13–15% of female patients); bicuspid aortic valve (50%); cerebral berry aneurysms.

Case
60

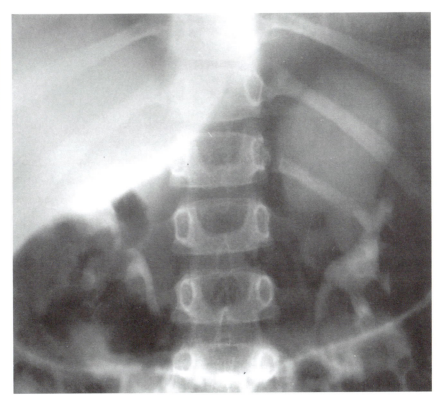

IVU of a child.

Question

61   What is the most likely diagnosis?
- ☐ **A**   Renal cyst
- ☐ **B**   Wilms' tumour
- ☐ **C**   Duplex kidney
- ☐ **D**   Staghorn calculus.

Answer overleaf

Answer

61   C   **Duplex kidney.**

Discussion

The IVU demonstrates an enlarged left kidney. The calyces, pelvis and ureter of the lower part of the kidney are seen clearly. However the upper part shows a rounded area of opacification but loss of the definition of the collecting system. This appearance is due to duplication of the left renal pelvis. The lower pole moiety can be seen to fill with contrast and the calyces and ureter are visualised, but the ureter which drains the upper pole is obstructed and the calyces and pelvis are distended in contrast fills.

Complete duplication occurs in 0.5–10% of live births and in 15–40% of cases is bilateral. The ureter from the upper pole moiety inserts below and medial to the ureter from the lower pole moiety and is subject to obstruction. A ureterocele is commonly associated. In the presence of a hydronephrotic upper moiety, lower moiety calyces may have a 'drooping flower' appearance

In some cases, the ureter may drain into the vagina or bladder neck.

The lower pole moiety is subject to vesicoureteral reflux and may atrophy secondary to chronic pyelonephritis.

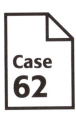

Case
62

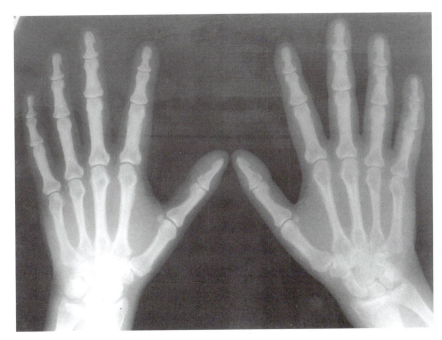

A 50-year-old woman with a history of thyroidectomy 10 years previously and now presenting with painless, swollen hands.

Questions

62a   What abnormality is shown?
- ☐ A   Finger clubbing
- ☐ B   Erosions
- ☐ C   Short fourth metacarpal
- ☐ D   Periosteal reaction.

62b   What is the diagnosis?
- ☐ A   Hyperparathyroidism
- ☐ B   Hypothyroidism
- ☐ C   Thyroid acropachy
- ☐ D   Metastatic carcinoma.

Answer overleaf

Case
62

Answers

62a   D   **Periosteal reaction**.

62b   C   **Thyroid acropachy**.

Discussion

Thyroid acropachy occurs in 0.5–10% of patients following thyroidectomy for hyperthyroidism, who may be euthyroid, hypothyroid or hyperthyroid. It mainly affects the proximal phalanges in the hands; less commonly the feet, lower legs and forearms are involved. The extremities may be swollen or clubbed.

Causes of bilaterally symmetrical periosteal reaction in adults include:
- Hypertrophic osteoarthropathy (HOA). Thick, irregular undulating periosteal reaction. It involves the shafts of tubular bones (especially the long bones of the forearm and leg), sparing the ends. Involvement of the hands is less common.
- Pachydermoperiostitis – a rare, self-limiting and familial condition that most commonly affects adolescent males. Compared with HOA it is relatively pain free. Periosteal reaction also affects the bone ends but otherwise has the same favoured distribution as HOA.
- Vascular insufficiency – the legs are affected almost exclusively. Phleboliths may be seen.
- Fluorosis – solid, undulating periosteal reaction. However, the bones are dense and ligamentous calcification is often present.

Case 63

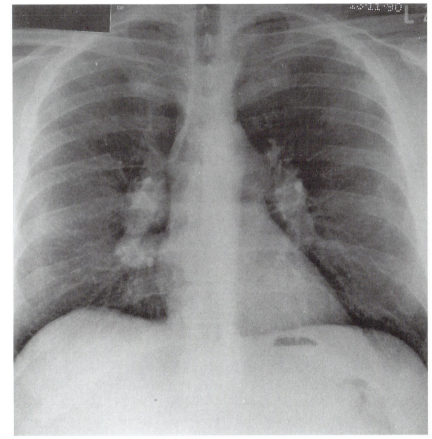

Chest X-ray of a 35-year-old man with a chronic cough.

Questions

63a   What is the main radiological abnormality?
- ☐   **A**   Hilar mass
- ☐   **B**   Asymmetric hilar lymphadenopathy
- ☐   **C**   Bilateral hilar lymphadenopathy
- ☐   **D**   Pulmonary metastases.

63b   What is the most likely diagnosis?
- ☐   **A**   Sarcoidosis
- ☐   **B**   Tuberculosis
- ☐   **C**   Bronchial carcinoma.

Answer overleaf

Case 63

Answers

63a C **Bilateral hilar lymphadenopathy**.

63b A **Sarcoidosis**.

Discussion

At clinical presentation the chest radiograph in patients with sarcoidosis may be:

- Normal (8%)
- Bilateral hilar lymphadenopathy (50%)
- Bilateral hilar lymphadenopathy + pulmonary infiltrate (30%)
- Pulmonary infiltrate ± fibrosis (12%).

Hilar lymphadenopathy is generally symmetrical and often accompanied by right paratracheal nodes. Rarely, hilar lymphadenopathy is unilateral (3–5%). Calcification of hilar nodes occurs in 5% of patients and can be punctate or 'eggshell'.

Lung parenchymal shadowing predominantly occurs in the mid and upper zones.

Other causes of bilateral hilar enlargement are:

- Enlarged lymph nodes:
  Lymphoma (50% in Hodgkin's disease). Generally asymmetrical, unlike sarcoid.
  Metastases. Generally unilateral.
  Tuberculosis. Rarely bilateral and symmetrical.
  Less commonly leukaemia, silicosis and viral infections in childhood.
- Enlarged blood vessels.
- Pulmonary arterial hypertension.

Case
63

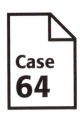

Case 64

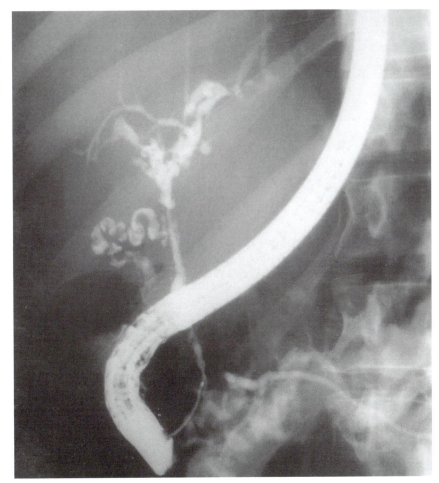

This is a 38-year-old woman.

Questions

64a   What type of study is demonstrated?
   ☐ A   ERCP (endoscopic retrograde cholangiopancreatography).
   ☐ B   Barium meal
   ☐ C   Cholecystogram.

64b   What is the likely diagnosis?
   ☐ A   Primary biliary cirrhosis
   ☐ B   Sclerosing cholangitis
   ☐ C   Cholangiocarcinoma.

Answer overleaf

Answers

    64a   A   **Endoscopic retrograde cholangiopancreatography (ERCP).**

    64b   B   **Sclerosing cholangitis.**

Discussion

Both the common bile duct and pancreatic duct are filled with contrast. There are multiple strictures affecting the extra- and intrahepatic ducts with slight to moderate dilatation of the intervening duct segments.

About one-third of cases of sclerosing cholangitis have coexistent inflammatory bowel disease (usually ulcerative colitis).

Complications include biliary cirrhosis, portal hypertension and cholangiocarcinoma (12%).

Other causes of multiple biliary strictures are:
- Primary biliary cirrhosis – disease limited to intrahepatic ducts (unlike in sclerosing cholangitis which affects both intra- and extrahepatic ducts in 90%) and strictures are less pronounced.
- Cholangiocarcinoma – usually a short, well-demarcated narrowing of the bile duct and only very rarely multicentric.
- Recurrent pyogenic cholangitis – variable picture. History usually helpful.

Case
64

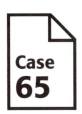

Case
65

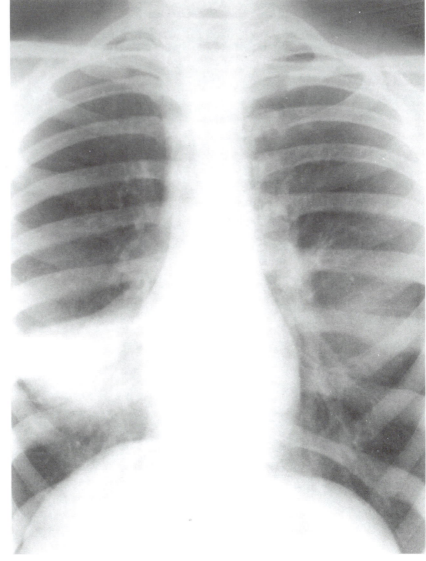

A young asthmatic patient presenting with a cough.

Question

65 What is the cause of this abnormal chest radiograph?

☐ A   Collapse/consolidation of the right middle lobe
☐ B   Collapse/consolidation of the right lower lobe
☐ C   Collapse/consolidation of the right upper lobe
☐ D   Carcinoma of the bronchus
☐ E   Lung abscess
☐ F   Empyema.

Answer overleaf

Case
65

Answer

65   A   **Collapse/consolidation of the right middle lobe**.

Discussion

Most probably secondary to mucous plug obstruction. The diagnosis is confirmed on the lateral film (Figure 65A).

In middle lobe collapse, the horizontal fissure and lower half of the oblique fissure move towards one another – best seen in the lateral projection. The right heart border is often obscured, particularly when there is associated consolidation. Since the volume of the middle lobe is relatively small, indirect signs of volume loss, including elevation of the hemidiaphragm, mediastinal or hilar displacement and compensatory hyperinflation, are rarely present.

Each lobe collapses in a characteristic fashion (Figures 65B and 65C) and radiological clues as to the cause of the collapse may be present, e.g. enlarged lymph nodes, bronchogenic carcinoma or an inhaled foreign body.

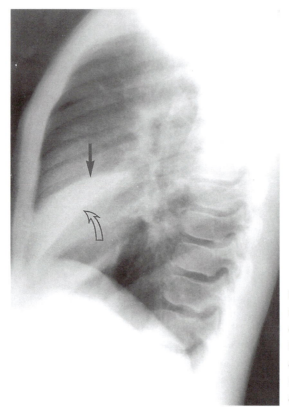

Figure 65A Lateral view – right middle lobe collapse/consolidation. Horizontal fissure (arrow) and right oblique fissure (open arrow) are approximated.

Case
65

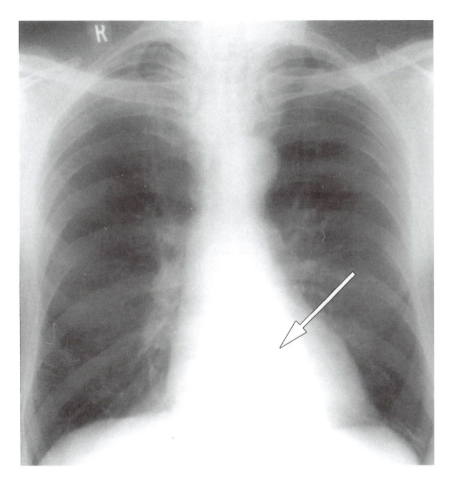

Figure 65B Left lower lobe collapse. Note the triangular density behind the cardiac silhouette (arrow).

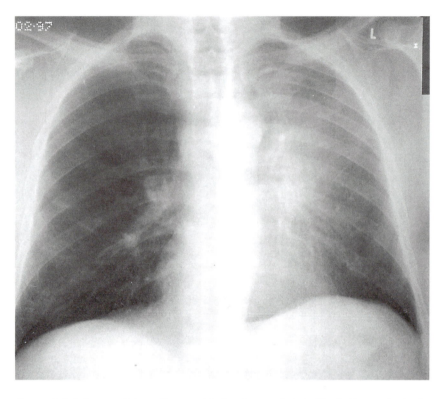

Figure 65C Left upper lobe collapse, with the characteristic 'veiling' effect and raised left hemidiaphragm. A left hilar carcinoma was the cause.

Case
65

Case 66

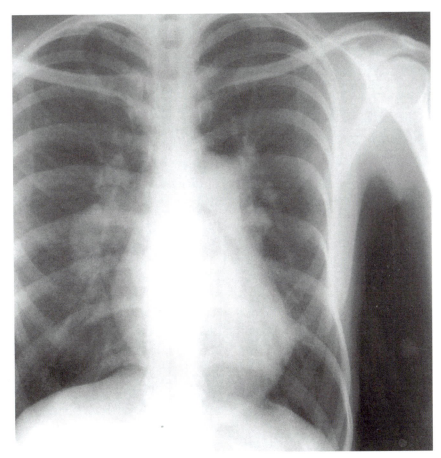

This 36-year-old man is cyanosed.

Question

66   What is the most likely diagnosis?

☐   A   Pneumothorax

☐   B   Pulmonary embolism

☐   C   Eisenmenger syndrome

☐   D   Coarctation of the aorta.

Answer overleaf   **Case 66**

Answer

66   C   **Eisenmenger syndrome**, due to atrial septal defect.

Discussion

The chest X-ray demonstrates dilatation of the central pulmonary arteries. The peripheral vessels appear 'pruned'. The heart is enlarged and the aortic arch is small.

The Eisenmenger syndrome refers to reversal of a shunt at whatever site, resulting from pulmonary arterial hypertension.

Chest radiograph appearances may provide clues as to the site of the defect.

With atrial septal defects (ASD) the heart size is often very enlarged with a small aortic knuckle (due to cardiac rotation) and the main pulmonary arteries may be markedly dilated.

With ventricular septal defects (VSD) the heart size is either normal or slightly enlarged and the pulmonary trunk is only minimally dilated. Distal vessel pruning occurs more gradually than ASD. The left atrium will be enlarged, but in many cases the chest radiograph appears normal.

Eisenmenger syndrome occurs in 2% of large VSDs by 2 years of age.

In ductus arteriosus defects, cardiac size mimics VSD, but the aortic knuckle is generally enlarged.

Causes of a small aortic arch are:
• Decreased cardiac output, e.g. mitral stenosis.
• ASD (left to right intracardiac shunt).
• Coarctation – long segment 'infantile type'.

Case
66

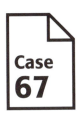

Case 67

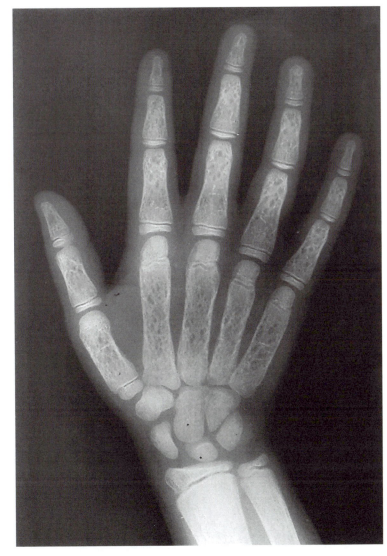

Hand X-ray of a 12-year-old boy.

Question

67   What is the most likely diagnosis?

☐   A   Thalassaemia trait
☐   B   Thalassaemia major
☐   C   Sickle cell trait
☐   D   Sickle cell disease.

Answer

67   B   **Thalassaemia major.**

Discussion

Marrow hyperplasia destroys many of the medullary trabeculae and expands and thins the overlying cortex. In children, this process is especially evident in the hands, when the shafts of the phalanges and metacarpals become biconvex instead of biconcave.

Other radiological abnormalities seen in thalassaemia major are:
- Skull – (Figure 67A) widening of the diploic space, thinning of the outer table and a 'hair-on-end' appearance. Involvement of the facial bones produces obliteration of the paranasal sinuses and mastoid air cells, as well as lateral displacement of the orbits.
- Chest – cardiac enlargement and congestive cardiac failure. Paravertebral masses (= extramedullary haematopoiesis).
- Spine – osteoporosis, exaggerated vertical trabeculae and fish-shaped vertebrae.
- Ribs, clavicles, feet – typical changes of marrow hyperplasia.

Marrow hyperplasia is more pronounced in beta-thalassaemia than in sickle cell anaemia and facial bone changes rarely occur in the latter, an important differentiating sign.

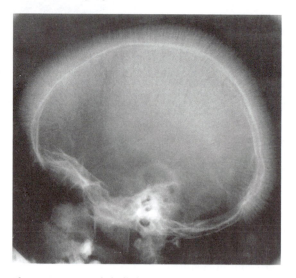

Figure 67A Lateral skull, 'hair-on-end' appearance. Note the normal calvarium inferior to the internal occipital protuberance (marrow content here is minimal). Poor pneumatization of the sinuses.

Case
67

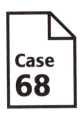

Case
68

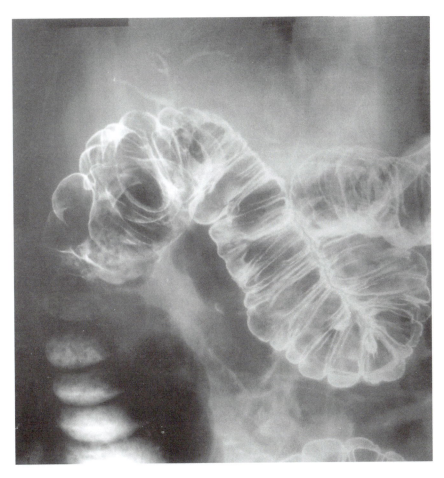

Film from a barium enema series.

Question

68   What abnormality is shown here?
   ☐   A   Barium is seen in the small bowel
   ☐   B   Barium is seen in the biliary tree
   ☐   C   Barium is seen in the peritoneum.

Answer overleaf

Answer

68   B   **Barium is seen in the biliary tree**, due to a biliary–colic fistula.

Discussion

Other biliary–enteric fistulae may be encountered:
- Cholecystoduodenal fistula (50–70%) – passage of a gallstone from an inflamed gallbladder directly into the bowel may result in a fistula; associated with gallstone ileus in 20%.
- Choledochoduodenal fistula (15%).
- Multiple fistulae (15%).

Aetiologies include cholelithiasis (90%), acute/chronic cholecystitis, biliary tract carcinoma, regional invasive neoplasia, diverticulitis, inflammatory bowel disease and trauma.

Abnormal barium filling of the biliary tree may be also seen after surgery, e.g. choledochoduodenostomy and with a patulous sphincter of Oddi on an upper gastrointestinal barium study.

Case
68

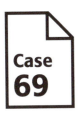

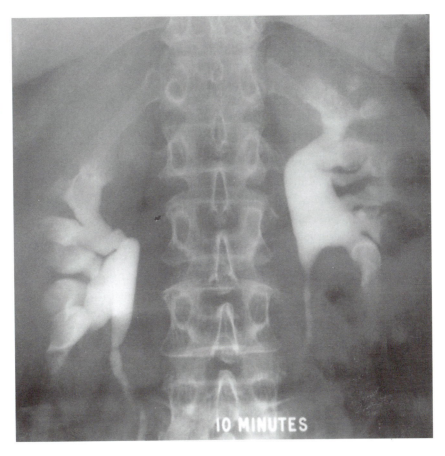

A 35-year-old female with a previous history of renal colic.

Question

69   What is the diagnosis?

- ☐ A   Chronic glomerulonephritis
- ☐ B   Chronic pyelonephritis
- ☐ C   Hydronephrosis
- ☐ D   Medullary sponge kidney.

Answer overleaf

Answer

69   D   **Medullary sponge kidney.**

Discussion

The plain film demonstrates enlarged kidneys and multiple areas of calcification within the medulla (rather than the cortex). The calcifications which are in the region of the papillae are said to have the 'bunch of grapes' appearance. Calcification on the plain film is seen in up to 80% of affected patients.

Medullary sponge kidney is a congenital cystic disease of the medulla resulting in localised dilatations of the collecting ducts in the papillae. Part or all of one or both kidneys may be involved and in 75% of cases the changes are bilateral.

Most cases are diagnosed on IVU: contrast examination characteristically reveals thick, dense streaks of contrast, 'bunch of flowers', radiating peripherally from pyramids. The affected calyces are often broader than normal and, similarly, the kidneys may be enlarged.

The differential diagnosis of abnormally shaped calyces also includes:
- Normal variant – 'papillary blush' – but without distinct streaks or nephrocalcinosis.
- Renal tuberculosis – calcifications tend to be more irregular and larger and strictures are usually evident.
- Chronic pyelonephritis – clubbed, dilated calyces with cortical scarring overlying involved calyces.
- Hydronephrosis – dilatation of the entire pelvo-calyceal system.
- Papillary necrosis – no distinct streaks.
- Congenital megacalyces. Renal size is normal. Calyces often appear multifaceted.

Case
69

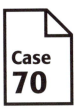

Case 70

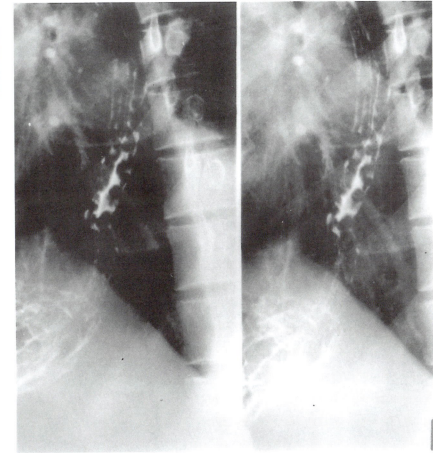

This is a barium swallow of a 32-year-old man with haematemesis.

Question

70   What is the most likely diagnosis?
- ☐ A Oesophageal carcinoma
- ☐ B Oesophagitis
- ☐ C Oesophageal varices.

Answer overleaf

Case 70

Answer

70   C   **Oesophageal varices.**

Discussion

Diffuse, round and serpiginous filling defects in the distal oesophagus, reflecting dilated submucosal veins.

The distal oesophagus is involved in portal hypertension. 'Downhill' varices in the upper oesophagus are due to superior vena cava obstruction.

Demonstration of varices does not necessarily establish the cause of haematemesis since one-third of such patients bleed from other causes, e.g. peptic ulcer. Endoscopy is the preferred investigation of choice.

Other causes of filling defects in the distal oesophagus are:
• Oesophagitis – can simulate the appearance of varices. Clinical details are usually helpful in differentiating. In oesophagitis there is usually a mucosal abnormality in addition to thickened folds. When due to reflux there is often also a hiatus hernia present.
• Carcinoma – fixed, thickened mucosal folds seen in the varicoid cancer form.
• Lymphoma – rarely presents as a submucosal tumour. Generally evidence of lymphoma elsewhere.

Case 71

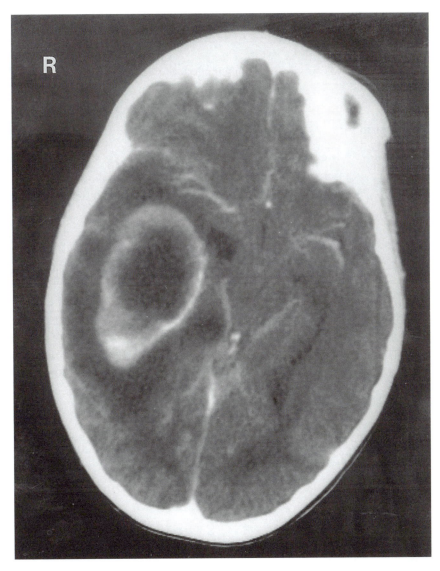

R

An enhanced CT head scan of a pyrexial 38-year-old patient.

Question

71   What abnormality is shown?
- ☐ A   Cerebral abscess
- ☐ B   Cerebral metastasis
- ☐ C   Glioma
- ☐ D   Intracerebral haemorrhage
- ☐ E   Cerebral infarction.

Answer overleaf **Case 71**

Answer

71   A   **Cerebral abscess.**
There is a ring enhancing lesion in the right parieto-temporal region with surrounding oedema and mass effect.

Discussion

The commonest causes of a cerebral abscess are trauma and direct extension from an infected sinus. In up to 30% of cases, abscesses are multiple. CT scanning shows a heterogeneous mass of low attenuation with oedema and loculi may be evident. Ninety per cent of abscesses show contrast enhancement, generally as a peripheral, thin, smooth ring. The relatively poor inflammatory response of deep hemispheric white matter may cause the capsule of an abscess to be better developed along the medial wall.

Other causes of cerebral ring-enhancing masses are:
• Metastases – irregular rim enhancement and typically located at the grey-white matter junction; multiple in 50% of cases (Figure 71A).
• Lymphoma – single or multiple ring-enhancing lesions.
• Glioblastoma multiforme. Thick irregular ring enhancement in a solitary lesion that tends to be situated in a deep hemispheric location. Rarely multicentric.

Note that oedema and also contrast enhancement may be suppressed by steroids.

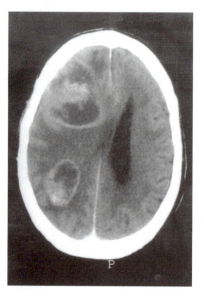

Figure 71A Multiple cerebral metastases from carcinoma of the breast. There is considerable associated oedema.

Case 71

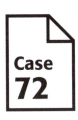

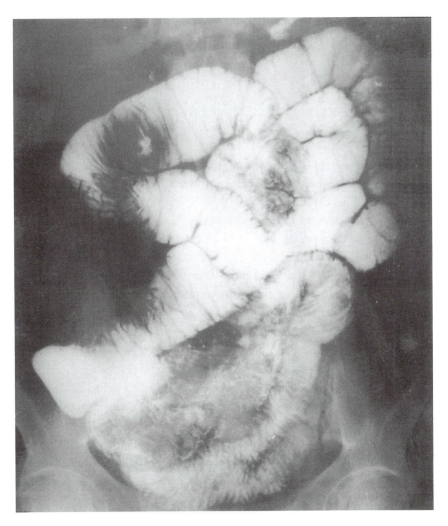

Small-bowel meal of a patient under investigation for longstanding diarrhoea.

Question

72 Which *two* abnormal features are seen?
- ☐ A Small-bowel dilatation
- ☐ B Large-bowel dilatation
- ☐ C Thickened bowel wall
- ☐ D Thickened mucosal folds
- ☐ E Filling defect
- ☐ F Perforation.

Answer overleaf

Answer

72 A, E **Small-bowel dilatation** and **filling defect**.

Discussion

There is small-bowel dilatation best seen in the mid and distal jejunum (normal calibre of mid small-bowel is less than 3 cm).

There is a large filling defect in the barium column in the mid jejunum (to the right of L2). This is due to the presence of a tumour.

There is flocculation of the barium – areas where the barium has a coarse granular appearance due to excess fluid in the bowel lumen. There is no perforation. The small-bowel folds are of normal calibre.

The patient has coeliac disease – gluten-sensitive enteropathy. Tropical sprue is the differential diagnosis.

In this patient with long-standing coeliac disease a jejunal adenocarcinoma has developed.

The radiological appearances of the small-bowel in coeliac disease and tropical sprue are identical and closely relate to the clinical state of the patient. Those who are most severely ill show the most severe small-bowel dilatation, which reverses with treatment. Small-bowel dilatation is seen in 70–95% of cases of untreated coeliac disease and is frequently associated with hypersecretion-related artifacts (break-up of the normal continual barium column and flocculation). Similar appearances may be seen in Whipple's disease, but there may be additional evidence of lymphadenopathy or bone changes.

A firm diagnosis depends on small-bowel biopsy. Coeliac disease is associated with an increased incidence of gastrointestinal malignancy (lymphoma 8%, adenocarcinoma of the small-bowel 6%, oesophageal and pharyngeal carcinoma).

Other causes of malabsorption with specific radiological features include jejunal diverticulosis, previous surgery, lymphoma and scleroderma.

Case 73

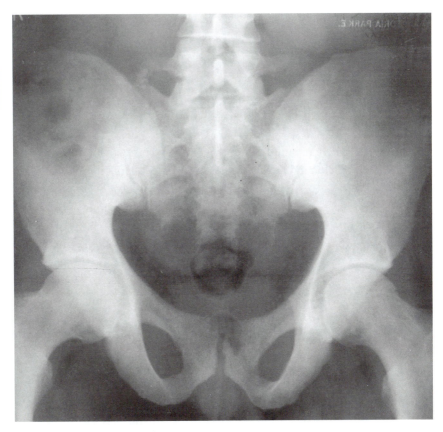

A pelvic X-ray of a 60-year-old male with anaemia.

Questions

73a   What is the main radiological abnormality?
- [ ] A   Decrease in bone density
- [ ] B   Increase in bone density
- [ ] C   Multiple lytic deposits
- [ ] D   Fractured neck of femur.

73b   What is the likely cause?
- [ ] A   Multiple myeloma
- [ ] B   Myelosclerosis
- [ ] C   Osteomalacia.

Answer overleaf

Case 73

Answers

73a B **Increase in bone density**.

73b B **Myelosclerosis**.

Discussion

There is a diffuse increase in bone density (osteosclerosis) with lack of distinction between cortical and medullary bone. There is also splenomegaly (the tip of the spleen almost overlaps the left iliac crest).

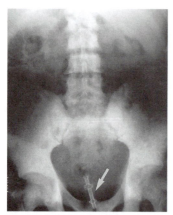

About half the patients with myelosclerosis have a widespread diffuse increase in bone density that primarily affects the spine, ribs and pelvis but may affect the whole skeleton. Uniform obliteration of the fine trabecular margins of ribs results in sclerosis resembling jail bars crossing the thorax. Extramedullary haematopoiesis causes massive splenomegaly.

Figure 73A Sclerotic bone metastases from prostatic carcinoma. Note the prostatic stent (arrow).

Other conditions causing a generalised increase in bone density include:
- Sclerosing bone metastases, particularly from prostate (Figure 73A) or breast carcinoma.
- Paget's disease. Characteristic bone expansion and coarse trabeculation also present.
- Renal osteodystrophy.
- Fluorosis. Calcification of ligaments is also often present.
- Osteopetrosis (Figure 73B). Rare hereditary bone dysplasia. The involved bones are dense but brittle and fractures are common. Characteristic 'bone within bone' appearance.
- Sickle cell disease. Additional features may include gallstones and step deformities in vertebral body endplates as well as avascular necrosis of femoral or humeral heads.

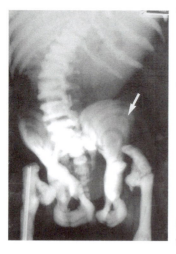

Figure 73B Osteopetrosis. Previous fractures, 'sandwich' lumbar vertebrae and 'bone within bone' appearances (arrow) are seen.

Case
73

Case 74

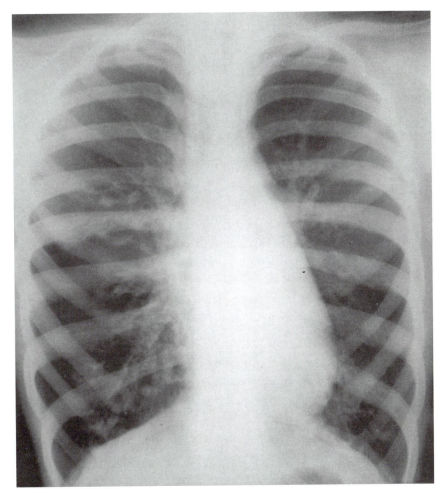

This 50-year-old man has haemoptysis.

Question

74   What is the likely cause?

- [ ] A   Carcinoma of the lung
- [ ] B   Bronchiectasis
- [ ] C   Goodpasture's syndrome
- [ ] D   Pulmonary oedema.

Answer overleaf

Case 74

Answer

74 B **Bronchiectasis.**

Discussion

Multiple ring shadows are seen predominantly in the mid and lower zones, some of which contain air–fluid levels. Ring shadows represent dilated bronchi seen 'end on'. Bronchial wall thickening is also present.

Causes of bronchiectasis include:
- Childhood infections – especially measles and pertussis.
- Congenital structural defects.
  Kartagener's syndrome (Figure 74A) – associated with immobile cilla, dextrocardia and absent frontal sinuses.
  Williams–Campbell syndrome.
- Immune deficiency states, e.g. hypogammaglobulinaemia.
- Secondary to bronchial obstruction – foreign body, neoplasm, mucous plugs (cystic fibrosis) and aspergillosis.

Thin section CT scanning is a more sensitive investigation for bronchiectasis and typically shows bronchi of greater calibre than their accompanying arteries.

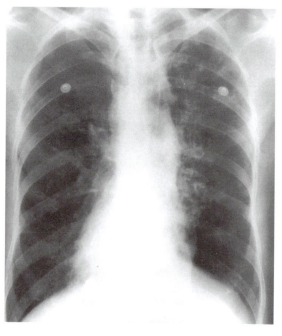

Figure 74A Kartagener's syndrome. Bronchiectasis and dextrocardia shown.

Case **74**

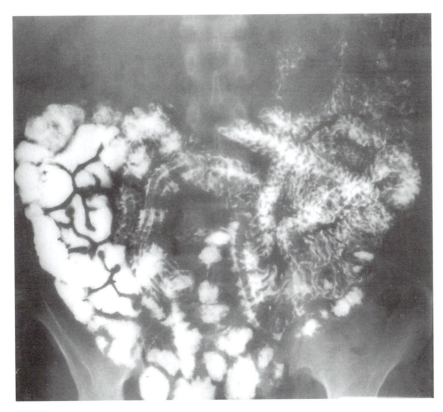

Case 75

This woman presents with abdominal pain.

Question

75   What is the cause?

☐ A   *Ascaris lumbricoides* (roundworm) infestation

☐ B   *Taenia solis* (tapeworm) infestation.

Answer

75   A   *Ascaris lumbricoides* (**roundworm**) **infestation.**

Discussion

Roundworm infestation is common in tropical areas but may be seen in any part of the world. The adult worm appears as a tubular filling defect in the barium-filled intestine. Within the tubular filling defect, a central thin thread of barium indicates that the worm has ingested some of the barium into its own alimentary canal. In children the worms may multiply, forming conglomerate masses which may give rise to intestinal obstruction. Trapping of gas between these coiled clusters of worms may cause a 'whirled' appearance or so-called 'Medusa locks' – which may be seen on the plain film.

The tapeworm (*Taenia solis*) may give a similar appearance but, unlike the roundworm, it has no alimentary canal and so cannot ingest the barium.

Case
75

Case 76

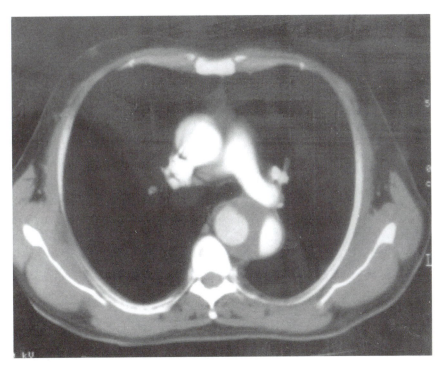

A CT scan of the thorax after intravenous contrast.

Question

76   What is the most likely diagnosis?

☐ A   Thoracic aortic aneurysm
☐ B   Abdominal aortic aneurysm
☐ C   Thoracic aortic dissection
☐ D   Abdominal aortic dissection
☐ E   Pulmonary embolism
☐ F   IVC thrombosis.

Answer overleaf   **Case 76**

Answer

76 C **Thoracic aortic dissection.**

Discussion

Two contrast-filled channels are seen in the descending thoracic aorta, where there is normally only one. Note the differential flow in the true and false lumens (i.e. different densities) in this type B dissection (confined to the descending thoracic aorta).

Additional signs that may be seen are inward displacement of atherosclerotic plaque by 4–10 mm from the outer aortic contour, left pleural effusion and pericardial effusion (particularly if extending into the ascending aorta).

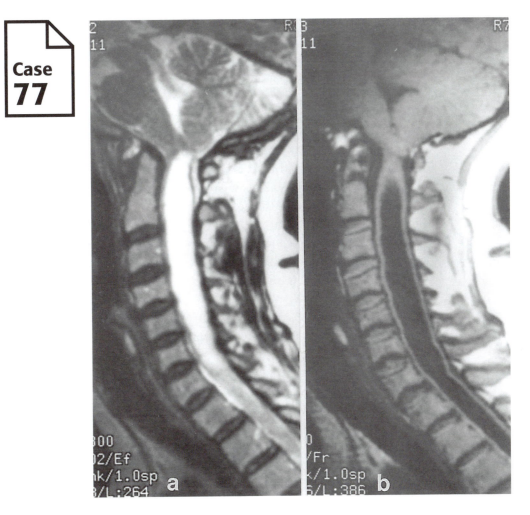

A sagittal MRI scan of the cervical spine, (a) T2 and (b) T1-weighted images.

Question

77   What is the diagnosis?

☐   A   Arnold–Chiari malformation

☐   B   Syringomyelia

☐   C   Syringobulbia.

☐   D   Multiple sclerosis.

Answer overleaf

Answer

77 B **Syringomyelia.**

Discussion

A cystic cavity is seen within the cervical spinal cord which is itself expanded. The cavity has discrete, smooth, well-defined borders and a uniform signal intensity which is isointense with respect to CSF (i.e. high signal on the T2-weighted image and low signal on the T1-weighted image). It extends from C1 into the thoracic cord, but the lower limit is not shown on these images.

In syringomyelia the cervical cord is involved most often and is enlarged in about 80% of cases. A widened spinal canal may be seen on plain X-ray in 30%, but the condition is best demonstrated by MRI. Extension into the brain stem = syringobulbia.

Between 70% and 90% of cases of syringomyelia are associated with cerebellar ectopia (Arnold–Chiari malformation), the cerebellar tonsils usually lying at the level of C1 or between C1 and C2. Other than congenital causes, it may result from trauma, inflammation (e.g. infection, subarachnoid haemorrhage, surgery) and tumours.

Low signal may be seen within the cavity on T2-weighted images due to CSF pulsations (flow–void phenomenon).

Case
77

**Case
78**

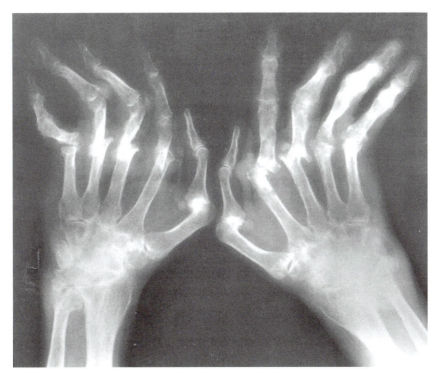

Question

78   What is the most likely diagnosis?

☐   **A**   Osteoarthritis

☐   **B**   Rheumatoid arthritis

☐   **C**   Psoriatic arthropathy.

Answer overleaf

Case
78

Answer

78   B   **Rheumatoid arthritis.**

Discussion

The X-ray of the hand demonstrates a bilateral, symmetrical, erosive polyarthritis predominantly affecting the metacarpophalangeal (MCP), proximal interphalangeal (PIP) and carpal joints.

At affected joints there is marked loss of joint space, bone resorption and soft tissue swelling. Subluxations are seen at the MCP joints, causing ulnar deviation.

There is periarticular osteopaenia.

There is erosion of the ulnar styloid bilaterally.

There is bony ankylosis of several PIP joints.

Other abnormalities that may be seen are 'swan-neck' deformities (hyperextension at the PIP joint, fixed flexion deformity at the distal interphalangeal [DIP] joint) and boutonnière deformities (fixed flexion at the PIP joint with hyperextension at the DIP joint).

Soft tissue swelling, joint space narrowing and periarticular erosions in psoriatic disease may simulate rheumatoid arthritis *but* psoriasis usually affects distal rather than proximal interphalangeal joints, is asymmetric and causes little or no periarticular osteoporosis.

Osteoarthritis predominantly affects distal joints and bones and density is preserved.

Case
78

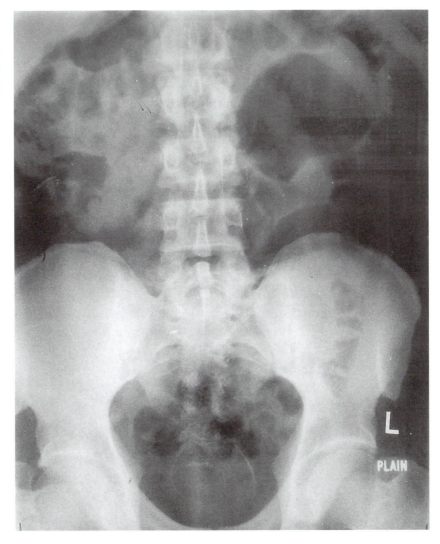

A 40-year-old male with haematuria.

Question

79   What is the most likely diagnosis?

  ☐   **A**   Carcinoma of the bladder

  ☐   **B**   Tuberculosis of the bladder

  ☐   **C**   Urinary schistosomiasis.

Answer overleaf

Answer

79   C   **Urinary schistosomiasis.**

Discussion

There is bladder wall calcification. Schistosomiasis is the commonest cause
of bladder wall calcification worldwide and is the result of infestation by
Schistosoma haematobium.

Thin, curvilinear calcification outlines a bladder of normal size and shape.
Calcification may spread proximally to involve the distal ureters (appearing
as two thin parallel lines) in 15%. Chronic infestation may be complicated
by squamous cell carcinoma of the bladder.

Other causes of bladder wall calcification are:
• Transitional and squamous cell carcinoma of the bladder. Radiographic
  incidence only 0.5%.
• Tuberculosis. Rare and usually accompanied by calcification elsewhere in
  the urogenital tract. Unlike schistosomiasis the disease begins in the
  kidney and spreads distally.
• Cyclophosphamide-induced cystitis.

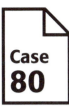

Case
80

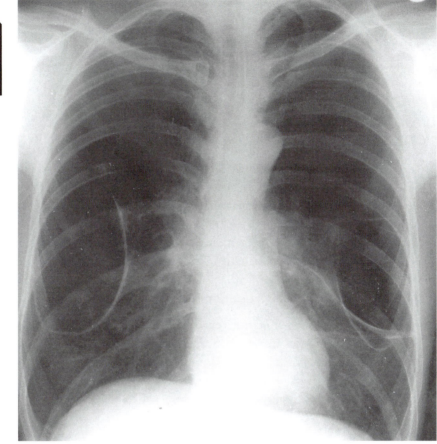

Question

80 What is the most likely diagnosis?

- [ ] A Alpha-1 antitrypsin deficiency
- [ ] B Emphysema
- [ ] C Bilateral pneumothoraces
- [ ] D Breast implants.

Answer overleaf

Case
80

Answer

80   B   **Emphysema** – predominantly affecting the upper lobes (most common distribution and associated with smoking). Bullae are present in both lower zones.

Discussion

The radiological findings ascribed to emphysema include:
* Hyperinflated lungs. The most reliable criterion is probably that of a low, flat diaphragm. In general a right hemidiaphragm that is at or below the anterior end of the seventh rib in the midclavicular line can be considered low.
* A reduction in the number and size of pulmonary vessels and their branches, particularly in the outer aspect of the lung.
* Avascular areas with curvilinear hairline margins, i.e. bullae.
* Secondary, right-sided cardiac enlargement.

When other conditions occur in emphysematous lungs, the radiological appearances are modified, e.g. with heart failure the oedema may spare emphysematous lung. CT scanning is a more sensitive way of detecting emphysema than plain chest radiography.

In alpha-1 antitrypsin deficiency (Figure 80A), the striking feature of the emphysematous changes is lower zone predominance; bullae are not a major feature.

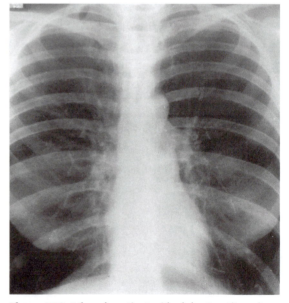

Figure 80A A female patient with alpha-1 antitrypsin deficiency.

Case
80

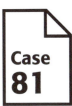

Case
81

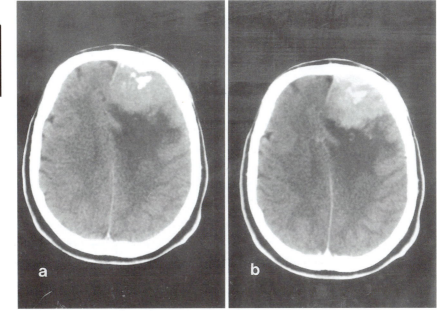

CT brain scans: (a) pre- and (b) post-intravenous contrast.

Question

81 What is the most likely diagnosis?

☐ A   Meningioma

☐ B   Extradural haemorrhage

☐ C   Intracerebral abscess

☐ D   Glioma.

Answer overleaf

Case
81

Answer

81   A   **Left frontal meningioma.**

Discussion

The CT scans demonstrate a well-defined left frontal, broad-based mass containing calcifications and of slightly increased density on the unenhanced scan relative to normal brain. Following contrast there is enhancement of the mass. There is also thickening and sclerosis of the adjacent skull vault. The low attenuation surrounding the mass in the left frontal lobe represents cerebral oedema. There is some midline shift from left to right.

A key feature of this lesion is that it is extracerebral and therefore the other options of intracerebral abscess and glioma cannot apply.

Meningiomas are solid, well-circumscribed, generally benign tumours that arise from the meninges, projecting inward from the dura and indenting and compressing the underlying brain.

These extracerebral tumours account for approximately 20% of adult brain tumours. Frequent sites of origin include the frontal and parietal convexities and parasagittal regions as well as the sphenoid wing, olfactory groove and suprasellar regions.

Multiple meningiomas occur in 6–9% and are associated with neurofibromatosis.

Typical CT radiological features of a meningioma include hyperdensity (± calcifications in 15%) pre-contrast (in 95%), adjacent bone thickening (90%) and striking homogeneous enhancement of the tumour mass.

Case 82

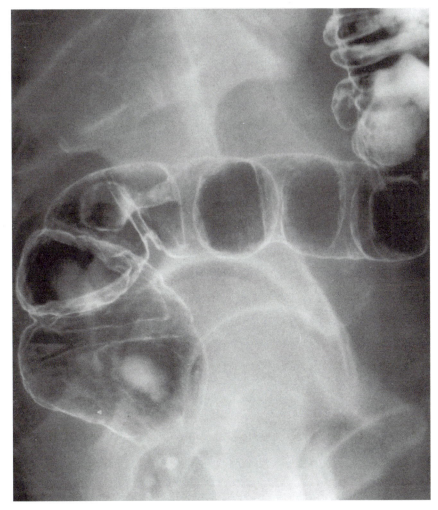

Question

82   What is the most likely diagnosis?

☐   A   Colonic polyp

☐   B   Colonic ulcer

☐   C   Small-bowel polyp

☐   D   Small-bowel ulcer.

Answer overleaf

Case 82

Answer

82 A **Colonic polyp.**

Discussion

A large, solitary, pedunculated polyp is seen in the distal sigmoid colon on this lateral view of the rectum from a barium enema series. Ninety-three per cent of colorectal carcinomas arise from adenomatous polyps and most commonly occur in the sigmoid colon (20–37%).

The malignant potential of a colonic polyp depends upon its size and degree of cellular dysplasia. Polyps measuring 5–9 mm are most likely to be adenomatous and have a 1% probability of containing invasive malignancy. Polyps measuring 1–2 cm in diameter have a 4–10% incidence of malignancy. Polyps more than 2 cm in diameter have a 20–40% incidence of malignancy.

Other signs of malignancy include irregular or lobulated surface, retraction (puckering) of the colonic wall and interval growth or change in shape. Double contrast barium enemas detect 82–98% of polyps greater than 1 cm in size.

Colonic tumours may have various appearances which include a discrete polyp, annular constriction or saddle lesion.

There is a 1% risk of multiple synchronous colonic tumours and a 3% risk of metachronous tumours.

Case
82

Case
83

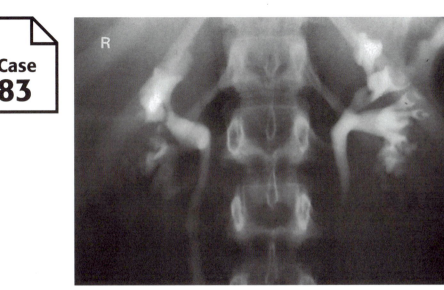

This 45-year-old patient has a history of chronic back pain.

Question

83   What is the diagnosis?

☐   A   Renal papillary necrosis
☐   B   Renal tuberculosis
☐   C   Chronic pyelonephritis.

Answer overleaf

Answer

83   A   **Renal papillary necrosis** – probably secondary to analgesics. Renal papillary necrosis is bilateral in 85% of cases with multiple papillae affected. Papillae show varying degrees of deformity which vary from long and thin to short and bulbous and includes cavity formation. A 'ball and cup' type appearance may be seen (as in the left kidney in this case).

Discussion

If total sloughing ensues, the sloughed papillary tissue may: fragment and be passed in the urine; cause ureteric obstruction; remain free in a calyx; remain in the renal pelvis and calcify.

Calyces appear club-shaped or round after the total sloughing of a papilla.

The causes of renal papillary necrosis include: *A*nalgesics aspirin; *D*iabetes mellitus; *I*nfants in shock; *P*yelonephritis; *O*bstruction; *S*ickle cell disease; *E*thanol.

ADIPOSE is a useful mnemonic.

However, diabetes, analgesics and sickle cell anaemia are the most frequent causes.

Renal TB   The urogenital tract is the second most common site after the lung. Evidence of previous TB on chest X-ray is seen in 10–15% of cases but less than 5% have active pulmonary disease. Extrarenal signs on the abdominal film (Figure 83A) include calcified granulomas in the liver, spleen, lymph nodes and adrenal glands and paraspinal changes of TB (discitis and psoas abscess). Renal manifestations are unilateral in 75% of cases and include calyceal deformities, stricture formation (pelvicalyceal system and ureter) and often calcified masses. Autonephrectomy may occur (small shrunken, scarred, non-functioning kidney ± dystrophic calcifications). Vesical involvement leads to a reduction in bladder capacity. Prostatic, epididymal and seminal vesicle calcification may also be seen.

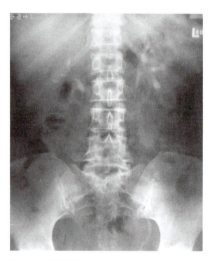

Figure 83A This case of renal tuberculosis demonstrates irregularities of multiple calluses of the right kidney.

Case
83

Chronic pyelonephritis   The calyces are clubbed and dilated. The important feature is that there is cortical scarring overlying involved calyces.

Medullary sponge kidney   May cause a similar appearance to renal papillary necrosis (see explanation to Case 69).

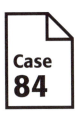

Case
84

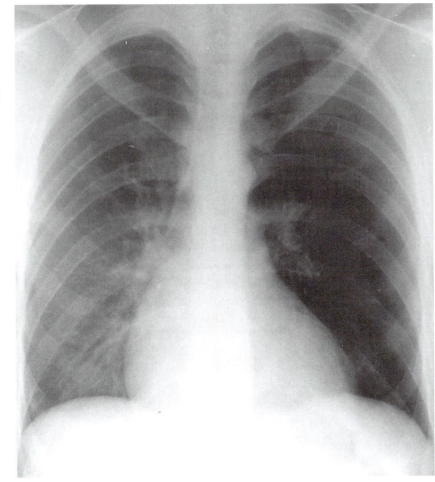

This is an expiratory chest X-ray of an asymptomatic male.

Question

84   What is the most likely diagnosis?

☐   A   Collapsed right lung
☐   B   Left pneumothorax
☐   C   Poland's syndrome
☐   D   Macleod's (Swyer–James) syndrome.

Answer overleaf   Case
84

Answer

84   D   **Macleod's (Swyer–James) syndrome**.

Discussion

This expiratory radiograph demonstrates a hypertransradiant left hemithorax with evidence of air trapping. There is small left hilum and reduced left pulmonary vasculature.

Macleod's syndrome is probably due to a childhood viral illness causing an obliterative bronchiolitis. On an inspiratory radiograph the abnormal, hypertransradiant hemithorax is generally of normal or reduced volume. Air trapping is seen on expiration.

It can be difficult in the presence of unequal lucency on a chest X-ray to decide which is the abnormal side. A useful rule is:
• If vascularity is decreased, the lung is abnormal.
• If vascularity is normal or increased, the lung is probably normal.

Causes of a unilateral hypertransradiant hemithorax include:
• Patient rotation (commonest cause). Check that the trachea is midway between the medial ends of the clavicles.
• Chest wall abnormalities, including mastectomy, Poland's syndrome (unilateral congenital absence of pectoral muscles) and poliomyelitis. Note that the vasculature will be normal.
• Pneumothorax: look for the lung edge.
• Pulmonary embolus: to a major pulmonary artery.
• Lung: obstructive emphysema (e.g. an inhaled foreign body), congenital lobar emphysema (most commonly the left upper lobe), unilateral bullae and Macleod's syndome.

NB. Exclude contralateral increased density, e.g. pleural effusion in a supine patient, or pleural thickening.

Case
84

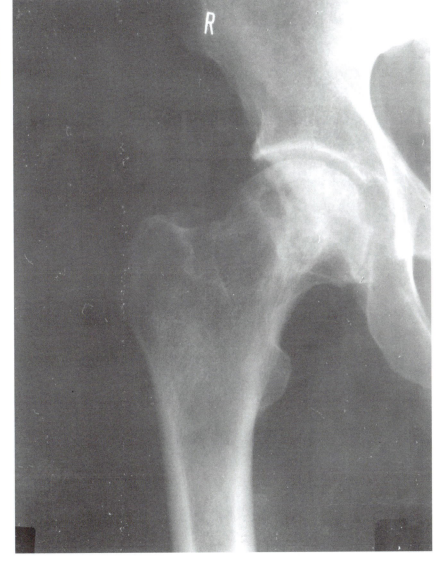

This radiograph is of a 45-year-old male.

Question

85   What is the patient likely to have suffered from?
- ☐ A   Congenital dislocation of the hip
- ☐ B   Avascular necrosis of the femoral head (AVN)
- ☐ C   Fractured neck of femur.

Answer

85   B   **Avascular necrosis of the femoral head (AVN).**

Discussion

There is patchy sclerosis throughout the flattened femoral head and narrowing of the joint space. These are the features of avascular necrosis of the femoral head.

The hip is the most common site involved in AVN, the hallmark of which is increased bone density at an otherwise normal joint. Radiological changes may take several weeks to appear and, in addition, include subchondral lucency, sclerosis, collapse of the articular surface and joint fragmentation.

MRI plays a valuable role in the early diagnosis of AVN (Figure 85A) and is more sensitive than radionuclide scans.

Causes of AVN include:
caisson disease, sickle cell disease, steroids, radiation, trauma, idiopathic (Perthes' disease), collagen vascular disorders, infection, and alcoholism.

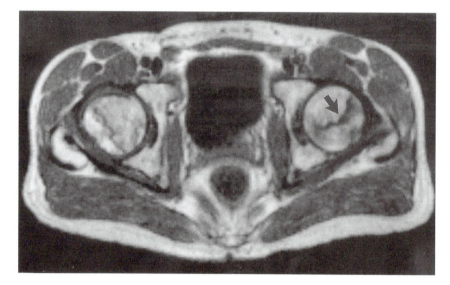

Figure 85A MRI scan (axial) T1-weighted image showing typical findings of AVN affecting both hips. Note the serpiginous cleft of low signal intensity (arrow) giving the appearance of 'tennis balls'.

Case
85

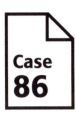

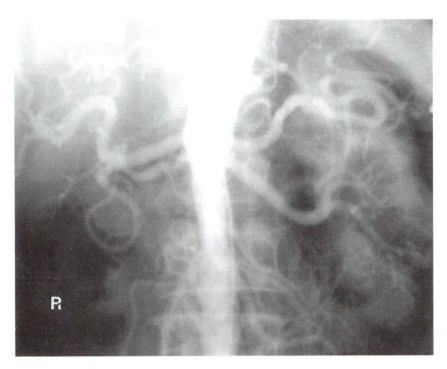

This 55-year-old man has hypertension.

Question

86   What is the likely cause?

☐   A   Polyarteritis nodosa
☐   B   Renal artery stenosis
☐   C   Fibromuscular dysplasia
☐   D   Polycystic renal disease.

Answer overleaf

Answer

86   B   **Right renal artery stenosis.**

Discussion

Arteriosclerosis is responsible for two-thirds of renovascular causes of hypertension and typically affects the proximal 2 cm of the renal artery. It is more common in men.

This is in contrast to fibromuscular dysplasia, responsible for one-third of renovascular causes of hypertension, which mainly affects women under the age of 40 and occurs in the mid and distal renal artery, sparing the proximal third of the main renal artery in 98% of cases. It is bilateral in 60% of cases and, if alternating areas of stenoses and dilatations are present (60–70%), a 'string of beads' appearance occurs.

The signs of unilateral renal artery stenosis on IVU are:
• A small smooth kidney.
• Unilateral delay of 1 minute or more in the appearance of opacified calyces.
• Increased density of opacified calyces.
• Ureteric notching by collateral vessels.

Polyarteritis nodosa is a systemic connective tissue disorder characterised by focal areas of necrotising arteritis with aneurysm formation. A renal angiogram shows characteristic 1–5 mm vacular aneurysms typically involving small- to medium-sized arteries.

Case
86

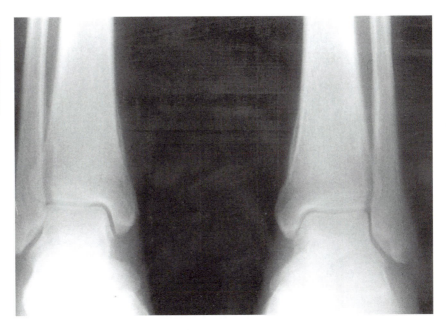

X-ray of the ankles.

Question

87   What is the cause of the abnormality seen here?

    ☐ **A** Osteomyelitis

    ☐ **B** Hypertrophic osteoarthropathy

    ☐ **C** Trauma.

Answer overleaf

Answer

    87 B **Hypertrophic osteoarthropathy.**

Discussion

Periosteal proliferation of new bone, at first smooth and then rough and undulating, is seen earliest along the distal third of the radius and ulna, then the distal tibia and fibula. Distal phalanges and the axial skeleton are rarely affected.

Radiologically, soft tissue swelling may be seen over distal phalanges if clubbing is present, but the underlying bone is normal and erosions do not occur. In the long bones, periostitis affects the distal diaphyses, but the bone ends are not involved. It causes a painful symmetrical arthropathy.

The vast majority of cases are associated with bronchogenic carcinoma, up to 12% of which have HOA, with the exception of oat cell carcinomas.

Of the benign causes, the highest incidence is found with pleural fibroma (Figure 87A).

Infection and trauma also cause a periosteal reaction, but this is localised.

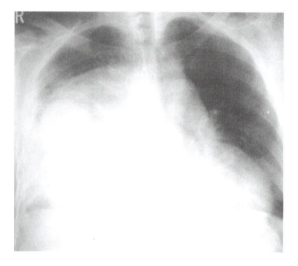

Figure 87A Large right pleural fibroma, causing mediastinal shift to the left.

Case
87

Case 88

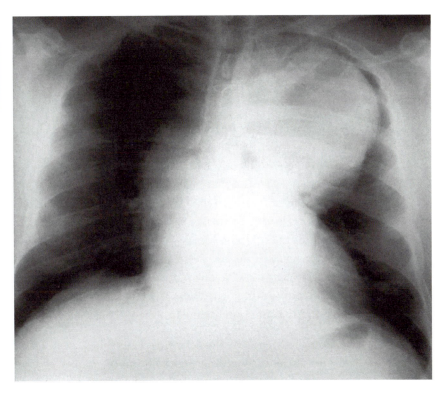

This young man is tall and thin.

Question

88   What is the likely diagnosis?

☐   A   Bronchogenic carcinoma
☐   B   Upper lobe collapse
☐   C   Lymphoma
☐   D   Aortic aneurysm.

Answer overleaf

Case 88

Answer

88   D   **Aortic aneurysm**.

Discussion

There is marked enlargement of the aortic arch on the chest radiograph of this patient with Marfan's syndrome. The large superior mediastinal mass is continuous with the descending aorta inferiorly, and appearances are consistent with an aortic aneurysm (confirmed on CT – Figure 88A). Median sternotomy wires reflect a previous attempt at repair.

Other causes of an enlarged aortic arch are hypertension (which by itself only leads to slight unfolding, with left ventricular enlargement), aortic incompetence (prominent ascending aorta) and aortic stenosis (poststenotic dilatation ± aortic valve calcification).

Unfolding of the aorta often gives the impression of an enlarged aortic arch and is a common finding in elderly people.

Aetiologies of thoracic aortic aneurysm include:
- Atherosclerosis – prominent calcification.
- Trauma.
- Infection, e.g. syphilitic aortitis, subacute bacterial endocarditis.
- Intrinsic abnormality, e.g. Marfan's syndrome.

The mass is continuous with the aorta and it involves the superior and posterior mediastinum. Other mediastinal masses may cause a similar appearance such as lymphoma (anterior mediastinum) and bronchogenic carcinoma may cause a large mass vented on the hilum.

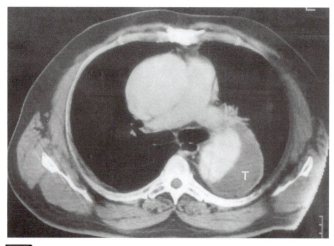

Figure 88A Contrast-enhanced CT of the thorax showing a large aortic aneurysm involving both the ascending and descending thoracic aorta. Note the eccentric thrombus (T) in the descending aorta.

Case
88

Case
89

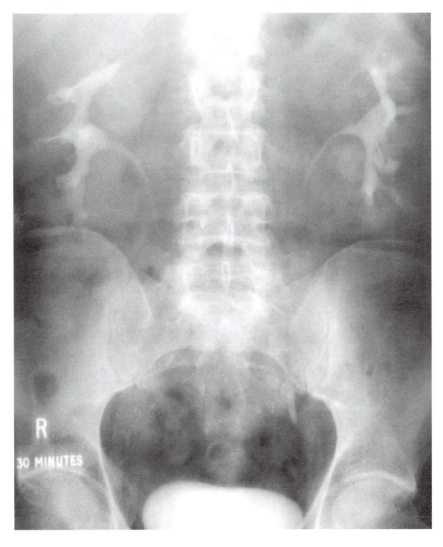

IVU in a patient with hypertension.

Questions

89a Name *two* features seen here?
- ☐ A Large kidneys
- ☐ B Small kidneys
- ☐ C Distortion of the collecting system
- ☐ D Dilatation of the collecting system.

89b What is the likely diagnosis?
- ☐ A Polycystic kidney disease
- ☐ B Polyarteritis nodosa
- ☐ C Renal cell carcinoma.

Answer overleaf

Case
89

Answers

89a A, C **Large kidneys** with **distortion of the collecting system**.

89b A **Polycystic kidney disease**.

Discussion

The IVU shows that both kidneys are enlarged (normal renal size approximates to the length of three vertebral bodies and their discs) and there is marked distortion of the collecting systems caused by the multiple cysts.

Associations include:
- Cysts in the liver (25–50%) and pancreas (9%).
- Saccular berry aneurysms of cerebral arteries (10–30%).

This appearance is easily distinguished from other causes of large kidneys including renal infiltration (lymphoma, amyloid), urine outflow obstruction (hydronephrosis), interstitial fluid accumulation (renal vein thrombosis, acute tubular necrosis) and proliferative disorders (acute glomerulonephritis).

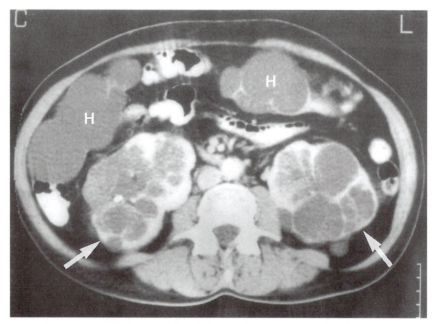

Figure 89A Enhanced CT scan of the abdomen showing polycystic kidneys (arrows) and multiple hepatic cysts (H).

Case
89

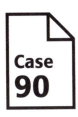

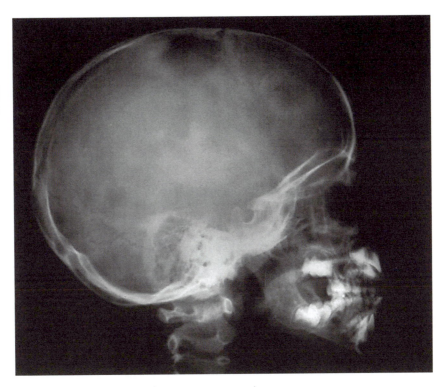

Skull X-ray of a 25-year-old patient with a chronic condition.

Question

90 What diagnosis can be made from this X-ray?
   ☐ A Multiple myeloma
   ☐ B Langerhans cell histiocytosis
   ☐ C Acromegaly.

Answer overleaf

Answer

90   B   **Langerhans cell histiocytosis.**

Discussion

Two, large well-defined areas of bony destruction are present (one near the vertex and the other in the frontal region). Both have bevelled edges. The frontal lesion has a sclerotic rim (seen in spontaneous healing or after treatment).

Other radiological abnormalities in this condition include:
* Skeleton – 50–75% have solitary lesions. Long bones, pelvis, skull and flat bones are the most common sites involved. Punched-out lucencies in the skull vault may coalesce to give a 'geographical skull' and involvement of the mandible may produce 'floating teeth'.
* Lung involvement in <10% is associated with a worse prognosis. Honeycomb lung, often with spontaneous pneumothoraces. Mid and upper zones are predominantly affected and lung volume is normal or increased (a useful sign).

Case
90

Case
91

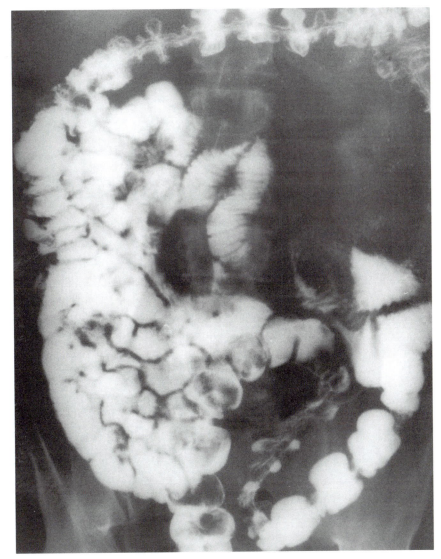

A small-bowel meal.

Question

91   What main abnormality is shown?

☐   A   Single stricture
☐   B   Multiple strictures
☐   C   Ulceration
☐   D   Cobblestone mucosal pattern.

Answer overleaf

Case
91

Answer

91   B   **Multiple strictures**.

Discussion

There are multiple strictures in the small bowel of varying length (Figure 91A shows an enlargement of a segment of jejunum) – due to lymphoma in this case.

The differential diagnosis for multiple small bowel strictures includes:
- Crohn's disease – indistinguishable from lymphoma, although there is usually additional evidence of altered mucosal pattern and ulceration (either longitudinal or transverse fissure ulcers or aphthoid ulcers). Strictures may be short or long, single or multiple.
- Tumours – including lymphoma (generally secondary to contiguous spread from lymph nodes), carcinoid and metastases.
- Tuberculosis – may be radiologically identical to Crohn's disease. Terminal ileum, caecum and ascending colon are often affected in continuity. Generally the stenotic lesions are shorter and the caecum more contracted than in Crohn's disease.
- Adhesions – history useful. Angulation of bowel which remains constant in site. Normal mucosal pattern.
- Radiation enteritis – typically in the distal jejunum and ileum. Absence of ulceration, cobble-stoning and asymmetry differentiates it from Crohn's disease.
- Infarction – progression is rapid, strictures tend to be long and ulcers are rare.

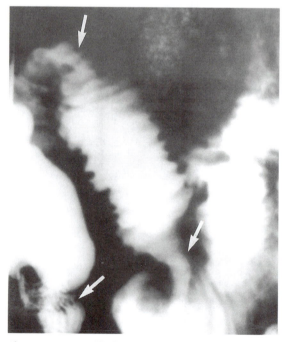

Figure 91A Magnified view of small bowel strictures (arrowed).

Case
91

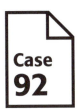

Case **92**

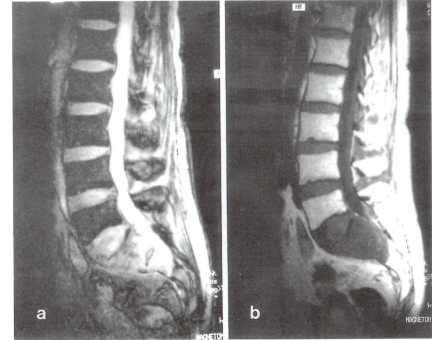

A 36-year-old woman with breast carcinoma. Sagittal T2-weighted and T1-weighted images of the lumbosacral spine.

Question

92   What is the abnormality?

☐   **A**   Discitis

☐   **B**   Metastastic deposit

☐   **C**   Primary bone tumour.

Answer overleaf   Case **92**

Answer

92   B   **A large sacral metastatic deposit is seen.**

Discussion

The bone marrow here shows marked alteration with low signal on T1-weighted images and high signal on T2-weighted images. There is extension into the L5/S1 disc space on sacral canal (note that the cord ends at L1 and it is incorrect to use the term cord compression below this level).

In adults, approximately 50% of all spine metastases arise from breast, lung or prostate cancer. All vertebral levels can be involved, although the lower thoracic and lumbar spine are the sites most frequently affected. Imaging findings – most metastases are osteolytic, although breast and prostate cancer can cause sclerotic lesions. Pedicle destruction is the most common plain film finding. Other frequent abnormalities include multifocal lytic vertebral body lesions, pathologic compression fractures and paraspinous soft tissue masses.

Bone scintigraphy is sensitive in the detection of metastases; only a 5–10% change in lesion to normal bone area is needed (which compares to 40–50% destruction needed for detection on plain films). However, bone scans are non-specific and may also be falsely negative in multiple myeloma, in which case radiographic examination is more sensitive for detecting osteolytic lesions.

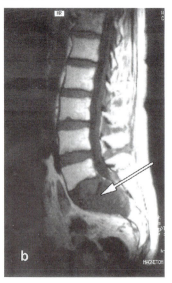

MRI is even more sensitive than bone scintigraphy in detecting vertebral metastases and exquisitely delineates cord compression, epidural and paraspinous soft tissue involvement. The most common pattern is multifocal lytic lesions, characterised by low signal intensity on T1 and high signal intensity on T2-weighted sequences.

Figure 92A

Case 93

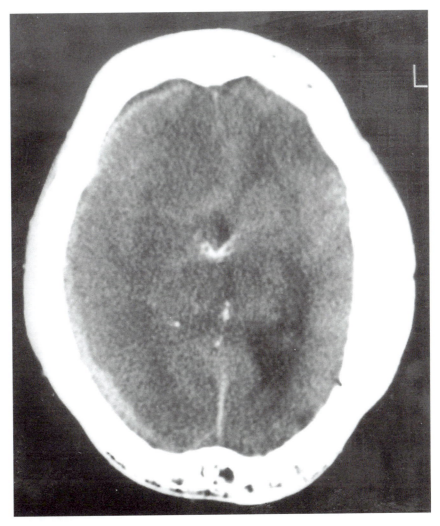

Unenhanced CT head scan of a 70-year-old man.

Question

93   What diagnosis can be made?

☐   A   Right acute subdural haemorrhage

☐   B   Left acute subdural haemorrhage

☐   C   Subarachnoid haemorrhage

☐   D   Extradural haemorrhage.

Answer overleaf   Case 93

Answer

93   A   **Right acute subdural haemorrhage**, causing mass effect, compression of the right lateral ventricle and shift of the midline from right to left.

Discussion

Subdural haematomas arise as a result of rupture of bridging veins and are seen predominantly in infants and elderly people and may be bilateral (25% in adults). Forty per cent of small subdural haematomas are missed.

Characteristically, there is an extra-axial, peripheral, high-attenuation crescenteric-shaped fluid collection. Concave inner margin and convex outer margin, following the normal contours of the skull vault, should be distinguished from the lenticular shape of an extradural collection. Extension of blood into the interhemispheric fissure also indicates a subdural location.

Density of collection changes with time:
Hyperdense (<1 week)
Isodense   (1–3 weeks)
   (see Figure 93A)
Hypodense (3–4 weeks)

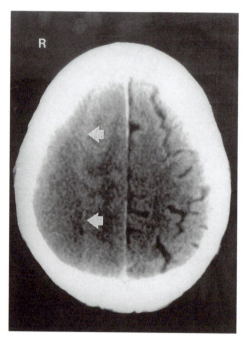

In most cases the subdural haematoma is accompanied by ipsilateral cerebral oedema and mass displacement.

(The skull vault shown in Case 93 is abnormally thickened as a result of Paget's disease.)

Figure 93A Isodense right subdural haematoma (the inner margins are arrowed). The skull vault appears artifactually thickened at this level, due to a partial volume effect from the vertex.

Case
93

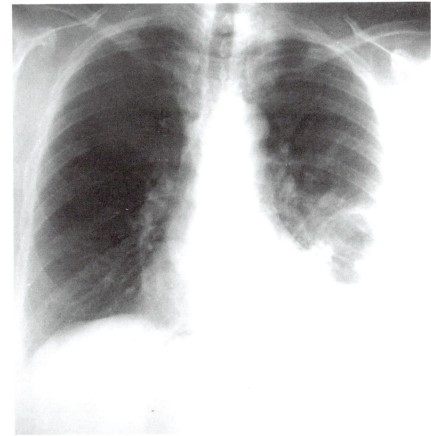

This patient has recently had a general anaesthetic.

Question

94 What pulmonary complications occurred?

☐ A Aspiration pneumonia

☐ B Left lower lobe collapse

☐ C Lung abscess

☐ D Pleural effusion.

Answer overleaf

Answer

94   C   **Lung abscess**.

Discussion

An ill-defined rounded mass is seen in the left lower zone in an area of consolidation (note the lack of visualisation of the left hemidiaphragm). The opacity contains an air–fluid level.

On the lateral view (Figure 94A), the air-fluid level is of a similar length indicating that the mass is spherical and most likely therefore to be a lung abscess.

The CT scan (Figure 94B) shows the abscess more clearly. It has irregular, thick walls; note the acute angle that its walls make with the adjacent pleura (for the differentiation from empyema see Case 112).

Causes of lung abscesses include:

- *Staphylococcus aureus* – thick walled, with an irregular lining. No lobar predilection. Associated with effusion and empyema. More common in children.
- *Klebsiella pneumoniae* – has a similar appearance, but favours the upper lobes and usually single.
- Tuberculosis – thick walled and smooth. Upper lobes and apical segments of lower lobes favoured. Usually surrounded by consolidation.
- Aspiration – a foreign body, e.g. tooth, may be apparent.
- Others – Gram-negative organisms, nocardiosis, aspergillosis, actinomycosis, amoebiasis and hydatid.

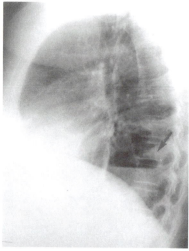

Figure 94A Lung abscess (lateral view), projected posteriorly over the dorsal spine (arrow).

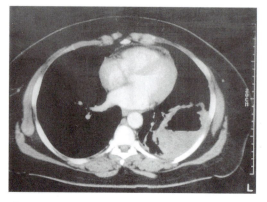

Figure 94B Contrast-enhanced CT scan – left lower lobe abscess with a thick, irregular wall.

Case
94

Case
95

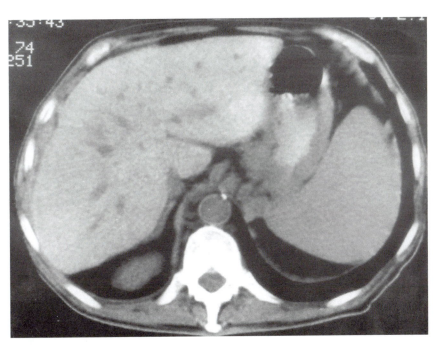

An unenhanced CT scan of the upper abdomen in a 48-year-old male with arthralgia and diabetes.

Question

95 What radiological abnormality is shown?

☐ A   Hyperdense liver

☐ B   Stomach wall thickening

☐ C   Pancreatic inflammation

☐ D   Hepatosplenomegaly.

Answer overleaf

Case
95

Answer

95   A   **Hyperdense liver.**

Discussion

A generalised increase in liver density is present. Note the increased discrepancy in attenuation between liver and spleen. Also the intrahepatic vessels are not normally visualised on a non-enhanced scan, but now stand out as low density against the high-density background. The liver density is similar to that of the oral contrast (iodine containing) in the adjacent stomach in this patient.

A diffuse increase in liver density pre-intravenous contrast may be due to:
- Haemochromatosis – there may be additional features of cirrhosis, portal hypertension or an associated hepatoma.
- Iron overload – e.g. from a large number of blood transfusions.
- Amiodarone treatment – contains iodine.
- 'Thorotrast' deposition – generalized (often inhomogeneous) increased density of the liver and spleen is caused by this previously used contrast agent. This alpa-emitting radionuclide has been associated with the development of hepatobiliary carcinoma and leukaemia.
- Gold therapy for rheumatoid arthritis.

This patient has haemochromatosis.

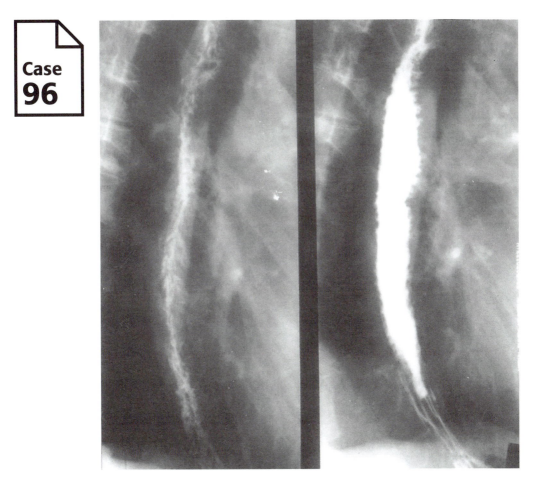

Case
96

This is a barium swallow of 40-year-old patient who had a previous renal transplant.

Question

96   What is the likely cause of his dysphagia?
    ☐   A   Oesophageal moniliasis
    ☐   B   Oesophageal varices
    ☐   C   Lymphoma.

Answer overleaf

Answer

96   A   **Oesophageal moniliasis.**

Discussion

There is extensive oesophageal mucosal irregularity with ulceration, producing a 'shaggy' appearance of the oesophagus in profile. The appearances are of oesophageal monoliasis.

This tends to occur in patients debilitated by malignant disease, diabetes, alcohol, renal failure, or by immunosuppressant, cytotoxic or steroid therapy. Identical appearances are produced by infection with *Herpes simplex*. However, gastro-oesophageal reflux remains the most common cause of oesophagitis, in which case a hiatus hernia is usually present.

Differentiation from oesophageal varices, which produce serpiginous filling defects in the barium pool, is generally easy (see Case 70).

Case
96

Case 97

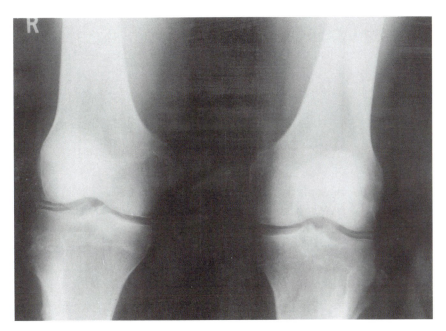

Question

97   Name *three* causes of this appearance.

☐   A   Rheumatoid arthritis
☐   B   Osteoarthritis
☐   C   Wilson's disease
☐   D   Haemochromatosis
☐   E   Psoriasis
☐   F   Gout
☐   G   Osteomalacia.

Answer overleaf

Case 97

Answer

97   C, D, F   **Wilson's disease**, **haemochromatosis**, and **gout**.

Discussion

The X-rays show calcification of the articular cartilage. The term used to describe this is chondrocalcinosis.

Chondrocalcinosis may be seen in:
*W*ilson's disease
*H*yperparathyroidism, haemochromatosis
*I*diopathic (ageing)
*P*seudogout (calcium pyrophosphate dihydrate deposition disease)
*A*cromegaly
*D*iabetes mellitus
*O*chronosis
*G*out
Mnemonic – *WHIP A DOG*

Chondrocalcinosis can occur in any joint but tends to affect the medial and lateral compartments of the knee, the triangular fibrocartilage of the wrist and the symphysis pubis. It is most commonly due to pseudogout.

Case
97

Case 98

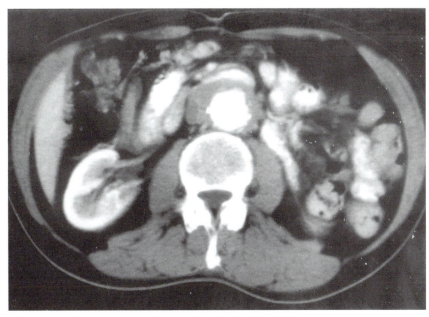

Upper abdominal CT scan with both intravenous and oral contrast. The patient is a 40-year-old male with back pain.

Question

98   What is the diagnosis?
  ☐   A   Aortic dissection
  ☐   B   Aortic aneurysm
  ☐   C   Lymphoma
  ☐   D   Mycotic aneurysm
  ☐   E   Retroperitoneal fibrosis.

Answer overleaf

Case 98

Answer

98   E   **Retroperitoneal fibrosis.**

Discussion

The aorta is of normal calibre but there is a mass surrounding it which has an attenuation similar to muscle. The appearance is of periaortitis, also known as retroperitoneal fibrosis.

Retroperitoneal fibrosis typically causes:
- Retroperitoneal malignancy (8%) – lymphoma and metastases especially from breast and colon.
- Inflammatory conditions – Crohn's disease, diverticular disease, pancreatitis.
- Drugs (12%) – methysergide, phenacetin, hydralazine.
- Aortic aneurysm.
- Retroperitoneal trauma and surgery.
- Idiopathic – 75% of all cases may be due to an immune reaction to atheromatous material in the aorta. May respond to corticosteroids.

Despite apparent ureteric obstruction, the ureters are often easily catheterised retrogradely, e.g. for stent placement.

Case
98

Case
99

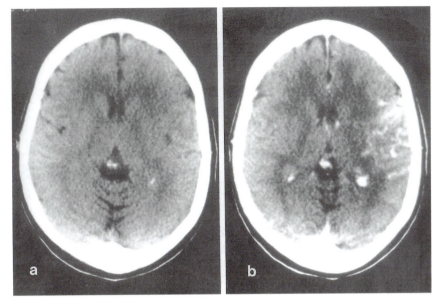

Pre- and post-intravenous contrast head CT scan of a 40-year-old man with seizures.

Question

99   What is the diagnosis?
☐   A   Meningioma
☐   B   Glioma
☐   C   Tuberous sclerosis
☐   D   Arteriovenous malformation.

Answer overleaf   Case
99

Answer

99   D   **Arteriovenous malformation (AVM)** – a congenital abnormality most often
supratentorial (90%) and commonly in the parietal lobe.

Discussion

No definite abnormality is seen on the precontrast scan. After contrast,
large, tortuous, high-attenuation structures are seen in the left parietal lobe
(representing serpiginous, dilated vessels), lack of mass effect or oedema.

An unruptured AVM may appear normal or only subtly abnormal on
unenhanced scans since the abnormal vessels are usually only slightly
hyperdense with respect to the brain and therefore difficult to identify.

In some cases, calcification suggests the presence of a malformation and
may be seen on a skull film (15–30%), as may prominent vascular grooves
due to the dilated feeding vessels. AVM may be complicated by
haemorrhage with a 2% risk per year of recurrent bleeding.

Case
99

Case
100

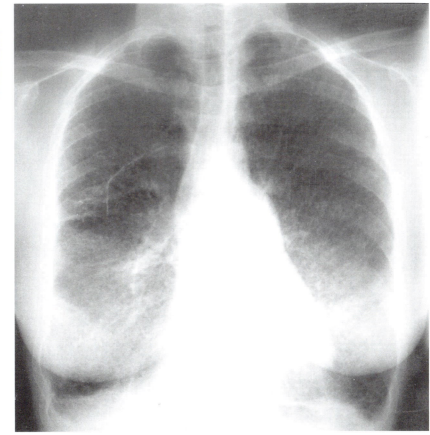

A 25-year-old woman.

Questions

100a   Which *two* features are seen on this chest X-ray?
   ☐   A   Upper lobe fibrosis
   ☐   B   Lower lobe fibrosis
   ☐   C   Increased lung volume
   ☐   D   Decreased lung volume
   ☐   E   Pleural effusion.

100b   What is the likely diagnosis?
   ☐   A   Tuberculosis
   ☐   B   Lymphangitis carcinomatosis
   ☐   C   Sarcoidosis
   ☐   D   lymphangioleiomyomatosis
   ☐   E   Asbestosis.

Answer overleaf   Case **100**

Answers

  100a   B, C   **Lower lobe fibrosis** and **increased lung volume**.

  100b   D   **Lymphangioleiomyomatosis**.

Discussion

On the chest X-ray there is a coarse reticular interstitial pattern which has a mid and lower zone predominance. The lung volumes are, however, increased. (Note the previous lung biopsy in the right mid zone where there is a line of sutures.)

Virtually all interstitial lung disorders are associated with progressive loss in volume (e.g. Case 51), unlike the following four conditions which are associated with a progressive *increase* in lung volume:

- Lymphangioleiomyomatosis: exclusively affects women of childbearing age. Characterised by an excessive accumulation of muscle in relation to extrapulmonary lymphatics. Recurrent pneumothorax (40%), large chylothorax (50–75%) and eventual honeycombing are seen.
- Tuberous sclerosis: radiographic appearances identical to lymphangiomyomatosis, including a high incidence of recurrent pneumothorax. However, chylothorax is unusual and other features, including epilepsy and adenoma sebaceum, are often apparent.
- Langerhans cell histiocytosis: similar radiographic appearances (occurring in < 10% of patients) often with a nodular component, but differing in that there is generally an upper lobe predominance. Recurrent pneumothorax is seen in 25% but pleural effusion is uncommon. Ninety per cent of patients are smokers.
- Neurofibromatosis: as well as the typical interstitial lung changes seen in 20% of patients and favouring the lower zones, other features are generally present, including rib notching, twisted 'ribbon' ribs, cutaneous tumours (appearing as nodules on the chest radiograph) and kyphoscoliosis.

Case
100

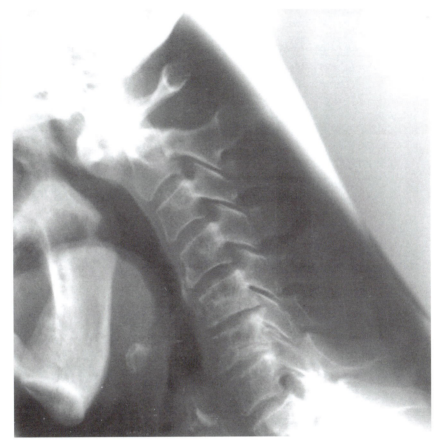

A preoperative lateral cervical spine X-ray.

Question

101   What abnormality is shown?

☐   A   C1/C2 subluxation
☐   B   C2/C3 subluxation
☐   C   Fractured odontoid process.

Answer overleaf

Answer

101   A   **Atlanto-axial C1/C2 subluxation** – diagnosed when the distance between the posterior aspect of the anterior arch of the atlas and the anterior aspect of the odontoid process exceeds 3 mm in adults or 5 mm in children.

Discussion

Atlanto-axial subluxation may be seen in:
- Rheumatoid arthritis: in 20–25% of patients with severe disease. Associated erosion of the odontoid process, as in this case, is often seen.
- Psoriatic arthropathy: in 45% of patients with spondylitis.
- Ankylosing spondylitis: in 2% of cases.
- Juvenile chronic arthritis: most commonly in seropositive juvenile onset adult rheumatoid arthritis.
- Systemic lupus erythematosus.
- Congenital disorders, e.g. Down's syndrome.
- Associated with a retropharyngeal abscess in a child.

Case
101

Case **102**

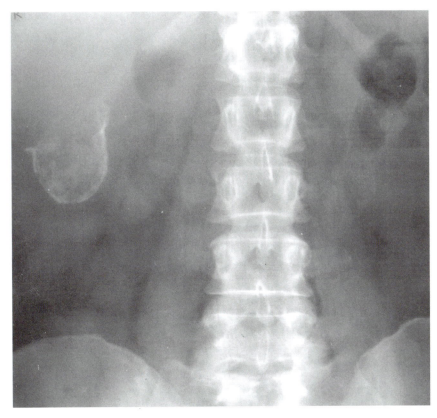

Question

102 What radiological abnormality is shown?

☐ A Staghorn calculus

☐ B Calcified gallbladder

☐ C Calcified adrenal gland

☐ D Calcification of the head of the pancreas

☐ E Haematoma.

Answer overleaf

Case **102**

Answer

102   B   **Calcification of the gallbladder wall** (porcelain gallbladder).

Discussion

Mural calcification around the perimeter of the gallbladder is found in 0.6–0.8% of cholecystectomy patients and is associated with chronic inflammation and hence the presence of gallstones (in 90%). The cystic duct is usually blocked. There is an increased incidence of carcinoma of the gallbladder.

Case
102

Case
103

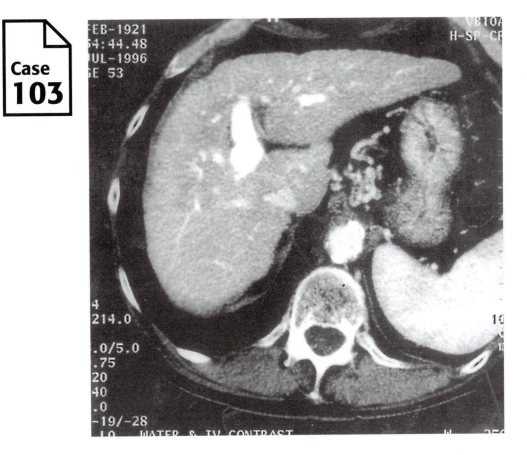

This is a contrast-enhanced CT scan through the upper abdomen of a 50-year-old alcoholic.

Question

103   What is the likely diagnosis?

- ☐   A   Liver cirrhosis
- ☐   B   Lymphoma
- ☐   C   Metastatic disease
- ☐   D   Chronic pancreatitis
- ☐   E   Hepatocellular carcinoma
- ☐   F   Alcoholic hepatitis.

Answer overleaf

Case
103

Answer

103   A   **Liver cirrhosis.**

Discussion

There is an irregular surface of the liver, compatible with cirrhosis (Figure 103A).

Anterior to the aorta (Figure 103B) there are serpiginous opacities which are varices.

Further images revealed splenomegaly (> 12 cm in length) and a solitary ring-enhancing rounded mass in the left lobe of the liver.

This mass (Figure 103A) is likely to represent a hepatocellular carcinoma given the clinical context of cirrhosis with portal hypertension.

Hepatocellular carcinoma (HCC) is associated with cirrhosis (most often due to alcoholism, hepatitis B virus or haemochromatosis) in 60–90% of cases. Approximately 5% of patients with alcoholic cirrhosis develop HCC which is most commonly a solitary lesion, showing enhancement during the arterial phase on CT scanning.

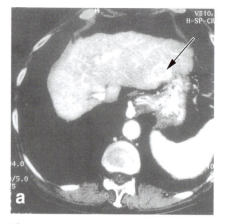

Figure 103A

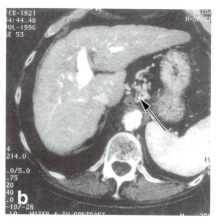

Figure 103B

Case
103

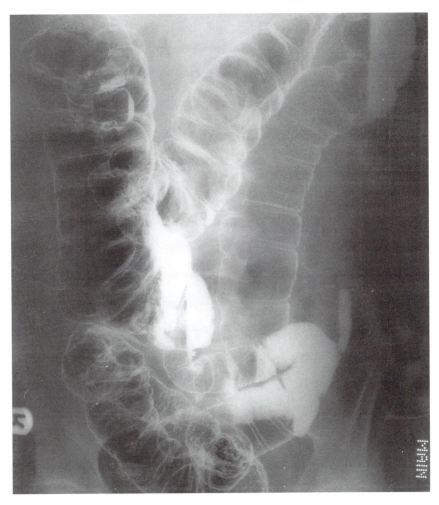

Barium enema of a patient with abdominal pain.

Question

104   What abnormality is seen here?
- ☐ A   Appendicitis
- ☐ B   Meckel's diverticulum
- ☐ C   Colonic polyps
- ☐ D   Small-bowel polyps.

Answer overleaf

Answer

104   B   **Meckel's diverticulum** – arising from the terminal ileum (projected over the left ileum).

Discussion

Meckel's diverticum occurs in 2% of subjects (most children <10 years of age) on the antimesenteric side of the ileum within 100 cm of the ileocaecal valve. It is the most frequent congenital anomaly of the intestinal tract; an outpouching of the rudimentary omphalimesenteric duct.

Presentation varies:
- Gastrointestinal bleeding due to ulceration of heterotopic gastric mucosa present in 30% of patients (60% in symptomatic children).
- Acute diverticulitis.
- Intestinal obstruction secondary to intussusception/fibrous bands/volvulus.
- Chronic abdominal pain.

Diagnosis may be made by an isotopic method following injection of 99mTc pertechnetate which is taken up strongly by ectopic gastric mucosa (sensitivity drops after adolescence), or by barium enema with reflux of barium into the terminal ileum. It is seldom recognized on small-bowel enema. Extremely rarely, it may appear as a large gas-filled viscus with a fluid level on the horizontal ray film.

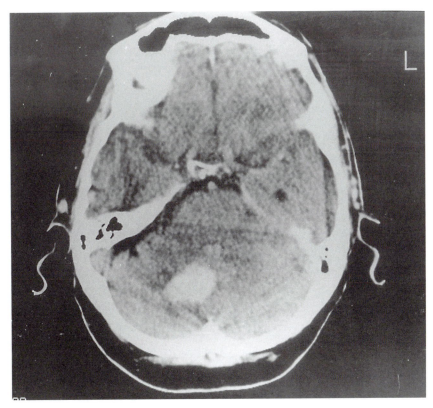

Unenhanced CT scan of the head of a 65-year-old.

Question

105   What is shown here?

☐ A   Acute cerebellar haemorrhage
☐ B   Subarachnoid haemorrhage
☐ C   Intracerebral abscess
☐ D   Intracerebral metastasis.

Answer overleaf

Case
105

Answer

105   A   **Acute cerebellar haemorrhage** (right hemisphere) with extension of high
density material (blood) into the fourth ventricle.

Discussion

In the majority of cases intracerebral haemorrhage occurs as a result of
hypertension. Less frequent causes include arteriovenous malformation,
aneurysm, trauma, vasculitis, anticoagulant therapy, tumour haemorrhage
(e.g. melanoma metastases, glioma) and haemorrhagic infarctions.

Blood can penetrate into the ventricles or subarachnoid spaces and give
rise to hydrocephalus.

The fresh haematoma is a sharply demarcated, round or oval focus of
homogeneously increased attenuation. The indirect signs of a
space-occupying lesion are often present. The density of a haematoma
decreases slowly, and is isodense with normal brain after 3–6 weeks, typically
resorbing from outside towards the centre.

Other causes of hyperdense cerebral masses on CT:
* Neoplasms: meningiomas (95%), lymphoma, metastases (30%) –
  particularly from melanoma, adenocarcinoma, renal cell carcinoma,
  bronchogenic carcinoma, glioma (10%) – most glioblastomas show
  mixed attenuation, ependymoma, medulloblastoma (80%), pituitary
  adenoma (25%), acoustic neuroma.
* Aneurysm.
* Colloid cyst (50%) – occurs in young adults, anterior to the third
  ventricle.

Case
105

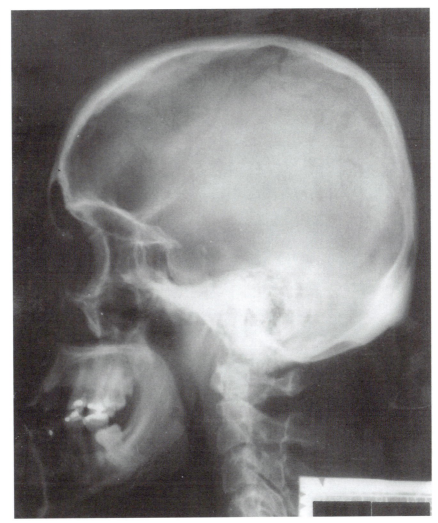

Question

106   What is the diagnosis?

- [ ] A   Acromegaly
- [ ] B   Hyperparathyroidism
- [ ] C   Multiple myeloma
- [ ] D   Paget's disease.

Answer overleaf

Answer

106   A   **Acromegaly**.

Discussion

The abnormalities shown are:
- Enlargement and erosion of the pituitary fossa.
- Prognathism (increased angle of mandible).
- Enlarged paranasal air sinuses and mastoids.
- Enlargement of the occipital protuberance.

Other effects of excessive growth hormone on the mature skeleton include:
- Vertebrae: an increase in AP and transverse dimensions with posterior scalloping in 30%. Kyphosis.
- Hands: 'spade-like' with broadening of the fingers (Figure 106A) and terminal tufts ('oak trees'). Widening of metacarpophalangeal joints due to cartilage hypertrophy.
- Joints: premature osteoarthritis and chondrocalcinosis.
- Soft tissues: increased heel pad thickness (>25 mm).

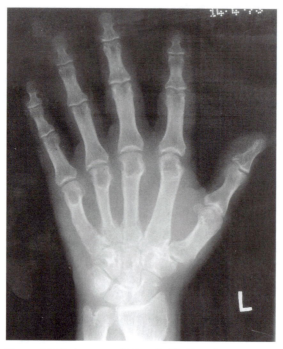

Figure 106A Acromegalic 'spade-like' hand.

Case
106

Case
107

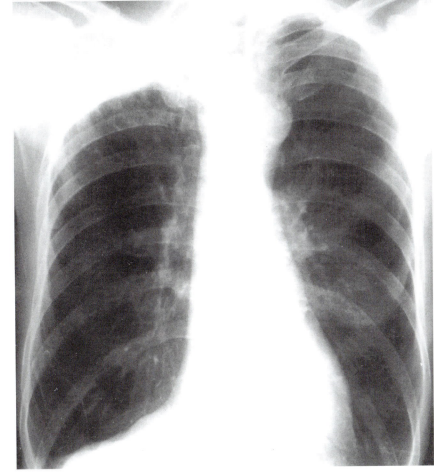

This 65-year-old patient has a painful right shoulder.

Question

107   What is the likely diagnosis?
- ☐ A   Loculated pleural effusion
- ☐ B   Pancoast's tumour
- ☐ C   Mesothelioma
- ☐ D   Plombage.

Answer overleaf

Case
107

Answer

107   B   **Pancoast's tumour.**

Discussion

Pancoast's original description included ipsilateral Horner's syndrome, due to invasion of the sympathetic chain, and local destruction of bone by the tumour, which may be of any cell type.

Radiographically, the tumours appear as a mass in 50–75% of cases and as an apical cap (resembling pleural thickening) in the remainder. Bone destruction is seen in one third of cases in the adjacent ribs or spine.

CT can be helpful (Figure 107A) for showing the full extent of the tumour, particularly chest wall invasion, although MRI provides superior information in this respect because of its multiplanar capability.

Another cause of apical opacification is plombage (Figure 107B). The lucite balls have smooth lower margins and there is often evidence of previous tuberculous infection at the other lung apex.

Although mesothelioma will cause a peripheral (plural base) mass there are no other features of asbestos exposure on this chest X-ray such as calcified pleural plaque.

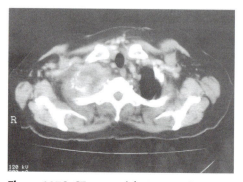

Figure 107A CT scan – right Pancoast's tumour.

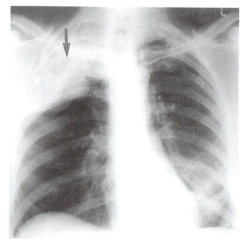

Figure 107B CXR. Plombage (arrow). Evidence of previous TB at the left apex; calcification, pleural thickening and upper lobe fibrosis with elevation of the left hilum. In addition there is acute, left basal consolidation due to a bacterial pneumonia.

Case
107

Case
108

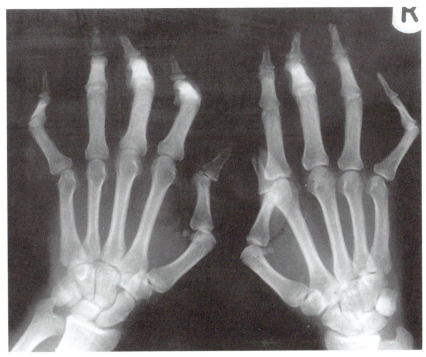

This 30-year-old woman has a chronic condition.

Questions

108a   Which *two* radiological abnormalities are seen on this X-ray of the hands?
☐   A   Joint erosions
☐   B   Phalangeal sclerosis
☐   C   Osteopenia.

108b   What is the likely diagnosis?
☐   A   Rheumatoid arthritis
☐   B   Osteoarthritis
☐   C   Systemic lupus erythematosus (SLE)
☐   D   Scleroderma.

Answer overleaf   Case 108

Answers

108a   B, C   **Phalangeal sclerosis** and **osteopenia**.

108b   C   **Systemic lupus erythematosus**.

Discussion

A non-erosive deforming polyarthropathy may be seen in SLE and after subsidence of frequent severe attacks of rheumatic fever (Jacoud's arthropathy.)

Other causes of phalangeal sclerosis are:
- Normal variant – 10% of the population.
- Rheumatoid arthritis – most commonly in association with erosive arthropathy.
- Scleroderma – in addition to soft tissue calcification, tuft resorption and joint erosions.
- Sarcoidosis – a lacy reticular pattern is often associated.

Case
108

Case **109**

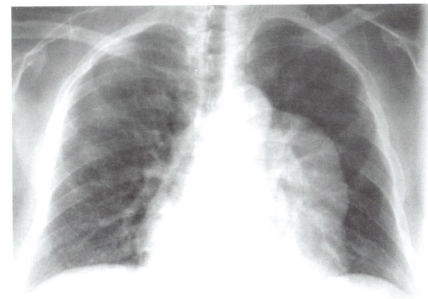

A chest radiograph of a 55-year-old male.

Questions

109a   Where is the abnormality located?
☐ A   Anterior mediastinum
☐ B   Posterior mediastinum
☐ C   Middle mediastinum.

109b   What is the likely diagnosis?
☐ A   Classic aortic aneurysm
☐ B   Pulmonary artery enlargement
☐ C   Thymoma
☐ D   Bronchogenic carcinoma
☐ E   Retrosternal goitre.

Answers

109a   A   **Anterior mediastinum.**

109b   C   **Thymoma.**

Discussion

There is a large, lobulated soft tissue density mass projecting to the left of the mediastinum. The descending thoracic aorta, aortic arch and left main pulmonary artery can still be seen clearly, placing the mass in the anterior mediastinum. No associated calcifications or pleural disease.

Thymomas are unusual in patients under the age of 20, occur in 10–17% of patients with myasthenia gravis and are usually benign. They are round or oval and smooth or lobulated. They may contain nodular or rim calcification or fat. They usually arise near the junction of the heart and great vessels (see lateral view, Figure 109A) and may protrude to one or both sides of the mediastinum.

A few are situated more inferiorly, adjacent to the left or right borders of the heart. They are best evaluated radiologically with CT.

Invasive thymomas (30% of cases) show spread beyond the capsule and metastases may be seen.

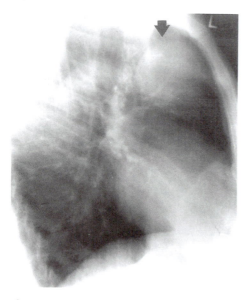

Figure 109A Lateral CXR. Thymoma (arrow).

Other causes of anterior mediastinal masses are:
- Lymphoma – enlargement of anterior mediastinal and retrosternal lymph nodes. There is often symmetric widening of the superior mediastinum on frontal views.
- Teratoma – usually larger than thymomas. Calcification and fragments of bone or teeth may be seen. More than 80% are benign.
- Retrosternal goitre – goitre extends into the superior mediastinum in 1–3% of cases and continuity with cervical soft tissues is visible. The trachea may be displaced.

Case
109

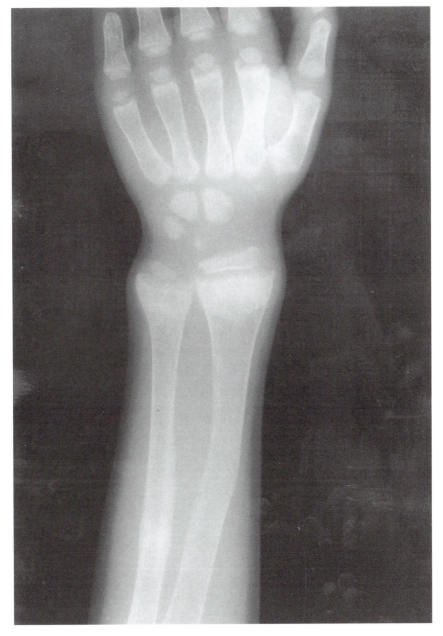

Question

110   What is the likely diagnosis?

☐ **A**   Rickets

☐ **B**   Osteomalacia

☐ **C**   Sarcoidosis

☐ **D**   Hyperparathyroidism.

Answer overleaf

Answer

110   A   **Rickets**.

Discussion

The abnormalities shown are:
- Abnormal metaphyses, with cupping and fraying.
- Generalised osteopenia.
- Bowing deformities.
- Looser's zone (mid-shaft of ulna).
- Soft tissue swelling around the wrist.

Radiological features are due to non-calcification of recently formed osteoid and to the effects of stress on the weakened bone and are most obvious at the wrists and knees.

Looser's zones are demonstrated less often in children than in adults with osteomalacia. Other features (in addition to those above) are rickety rosary (cupping of the anterior ends of the ribs), scoliosis, skull bossing and retarded bone maturation and growth.

Case
110

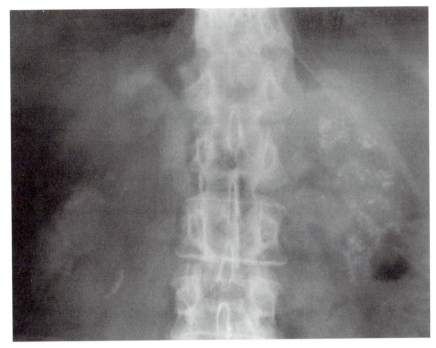

Question

111   In which condition may this abnormality be found?

☐   A   Polycystic renal disease

☐   B   Chronic glomerulonephritis

☐   C   Renal tubular acidosis.

Answer overleaf

Answer

111   C   **Renal tubular acidosis.**

Discussion

Renal parenchymal calcification (nephrocalcinosis) may be medullary – as in this case – or cortical.

• Medullary: the three causes above account for 70% of cases. Renal tubular acidosis is the commonest cause in children. Other causes include conditions producing hypercalcaemia or hypercalciuria, e.g. sarcoidosis, idiopathic hypercalciuria, hypervitaminosis D.

• Cortical: (5% of all nephrocalcinoses) – acute cortical necrosis, chronic glomerulonephritis and chronic transplant rejection.

Causes of more focal calcification include renal cell carcinoma, tuberculosis, hydatid disease and papillary necrosis.

Case
112

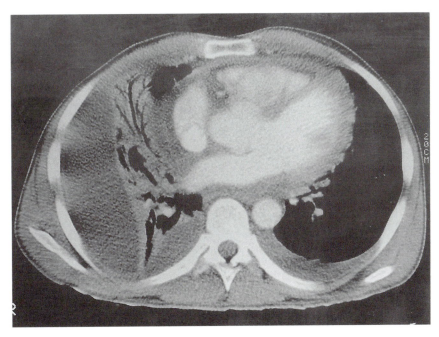

This patient has a pericardial effusion and a left-sided pleural effusion.

Question

112   What is the cause for the appearance of the right hemithorax (choose *two* answers)?

☐ A   Consolidation
☐ B   Lung abscess
☐ C   Empyema
☐ D   Pneumothorax.

Answer overleaf

Case
112

Answer

112   A, C   **Consolidation** and **empyema**.

Discussion

The abnormalities shown are:
- Pericardial effusion: fluid density within the pericardial sac (compare with the normal pericardium in Figure 94B).
- Left pleural effusion: fluid density within the dependent part of the left hemithorax.
- Right middle and lower lobe consolidation: (note the air bronchograms visible).
- A large right, lenticular-shaped pleural collection (predominantly in the lateral part of the right hemithorax, i.e. non-dependent aspect) – likely to be an empyema.

The distinction between pulmonary abscess and loculated pleural fluid can be difficult, but has important therapeutic consequences. Empyema requires early tube drainage, whereas antibiotics are given as first-line treatment in most cases of pulmonary abscess.

Features that may help differentiate between abscess and empyema are:
- Shape: loculated collections of pleural fluid tend to be based on the parietal pleura and are lenticular shaped or oval. If an air–fluid level is present, it will therefore be substantially longer on one view than in the other on the chest films. Abscesses tend to be spherical.
  In empyema the angle formed at the interface with the chest wall is obtuse compared with the acute angle more commonly associated with abscesses.
- Wall: the walls of an empyema are formed by thickened pleura and tend to be of uniform thickness and smooth ('split pleura sign'). The thickened pleura may enhance. The wall of an abscess is more irregular and tends to be thicker than in empyema and may contain dots of air.
- Adjacent lung: lung adjacent to an empyema is often compressed, unlike with abscesses. Adjacent pneumonia is unhelpful as it may be associated with both.

Case
112

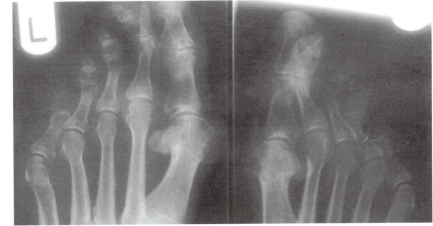

This 50-year-old man has swollen painful toes.

Question

113   What is the likely diagnosis? See also Case 2.
  ☐ A   Rheumatoid arthritis
  ☐ B   Osteoarthritis
  ☐ C   Gout
  ☐ D   Psoriasis.

 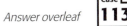

Answer

113   C   **Gout**.

Discussion

Asymmetrical soft tissue swellings around the first metatarsophalangeal and interphalangeal joints associated with asymmetrical 'punched-out' joint erosions at the joint margins (mostly set back from the articular surface). There is preservation of joint space and no apparent osteoporosis.

The distribution of affected joints and type of erosions favours gout.

The first metatarsophalangeal joint is the most common joint affected in gout (called 'podagra') and the classic history is that of recurrent attacks becoming more severe, frequent and polyarticular.

Radiological features are typically seen late (generally more than 6 years after the first attack) and include soft tissue swelling and 'punched-out' erosions which start near joint margins and have a classic overhanging margin in up to 40% and a sclerotic margin. Chronic tophaceous gout reveals eccentric soft tissue masses in a periarticular location (which rarely calcify).

Cartilage destruction (and hence joint space narrowing) is late and chondrocalcinosis occurs in 5% of cases.

The distribution of the arthropathy is usually asymmetric. The differential diagnosis includes rheumatoid arthritis which typically has joint space narrowing and osteoporosis and less well-defined erosions *and* psoriasis which has a predilection for the interphalangeal joints and does not have erosions that are as sharply defined.

Case
114

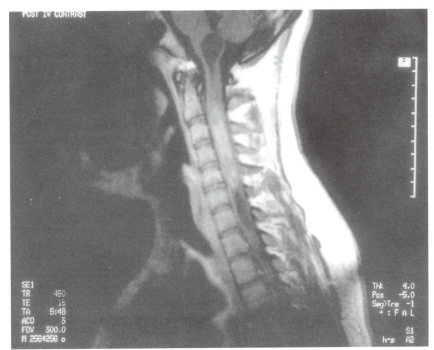

A T1-weighted, enhanced, sagittal MRI scan of the neck.

Question

114   What is the likely diagnosis?
  ☐   A   Multiple sclerosis
  ☐   B   Spinal canal glioma
  ☐   C   Spinal canal meningioma
  ☐   D   Epidural abscess.

Answer overleaf

Answer

114   B   **Spinal canal glioma**.

Discussion

The abnormalities shown are:
- Focal expansion of the cervical spinal cord (C1–C6) by a heterogeneously enhancing intramedullary lesion.
- A surrounding syrinx.

Appearances are those of an intramedullary tumour, most likely to be a glioma (in this case an astrocytoma).

Mass lesions in the spinal canal are classified as extradural, intradural and intramedullary in location.
- Extradural mass: prolapsed or sequestered intervertebral disc; metastases; neurofibroma; neuroblastoma; meningioma; haematoma; abscess; arachnoid cyst.
- Intradural mass: meningioma; neurofibroma; metastases; subdural empyema.
- Intramedullary mass: ependymoma (65%) – commonest in the conus and the lumbar region; astrocytoma (25%) – commonest in the cervical region. Appearance is similar to ependymoma; oligodendroglioma; Metastases – with lung carcinoma as the most common primary; lipoma – common in conus; haematoma.

Following contrast there is striking enhancement of most intramedullary neoplasms on both CT and MRI, although lesions are much better defined on MRI.

NB. The figures in brackets refer to the percentage of all intramedullary tumours.

Case
114

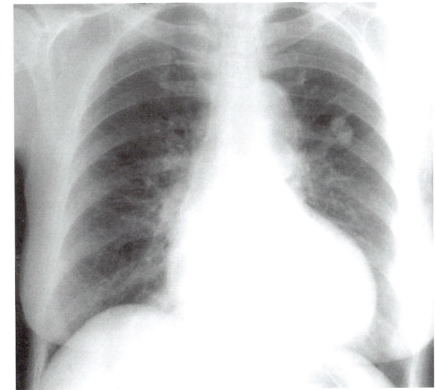

This patient has epistaxis and telangiectasia of the skin.

Question

115   What is the likely diagnosis?
☐   A   Pulmonary arteriovenous malformation
☐   B   Solitary metastasis
☐   C   Primary lung tumour
☐   D   Haematoma.

Answer overleaf

Answer

115   A   **Pulmonary arteriovenous malformation (AVM).**

Discussion

There is a sharply defined, lobulated, solitary, oval mass in the left upper zone with a band shadow connecting it to the left hilum.

Typical appearances of a pulmonary AVM – with the band shadow representing the feeding artery and vein. The history suggests that the patient may have Osler–Weber–Rendu syndrome with which the majority of pulmonary AVMs are associated and in which case they tend to be multiple.

The differential diagnosis includes other causes of solitary pulmonary nodules:

- Granuloma: secondary to tuberculosis/histoplasmosis. Well defined and commonly calcified and the most common lung mass.
- Malignant neoplasm: bronchogenic carcinoma (accounts for less than 15% of all solitary pulmonary nodules at age 40) and calcification is very rare, metastases (25% are solitary) and alveolar cell carcinoma.
- Benign neoplasm: adenoma (90% occur around the hilum) and hamartoma (may have 'popcorn' calcification and usually within 2 cm of the pleura).
- Infections: pneumonia, hydatid, abscess.
- Congenital: sequestration and bronchogenic cyst.
- Vascular: haematoma and pulmonary infarction.

Features that may help differentiate include:

- Spiculations – strongly suggestive of primary malignancy (90% of irregular, spiculated lesions are malignant), whereas 80% of sharply marginated lesions are benign.
- Calcifications – most suggestive of granuloma.
- Change in size with time – a rapid increase in size suggests malignancy.
- A vessel leading to a mass indicates an AVM or pulmonary varix.

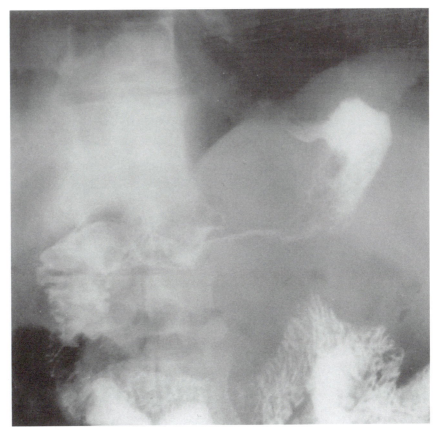

Small-bowel meal of a 70-year-old male with weight loss.

Question

116   What is the diagnosis?

   ☐ **A** Gastric carcinoma

   ☐ **B** Coeliac disease

   ☐ **C** Small-bowel obstruction.

Answer overleaf

Answer

116   A   **Gastric carcinoma** (linitis plastica).

Discussion

There is diffuse, irregular narrowing and contraction of the stomach, particularly in the antrum and body regions.

The appearance of gastric carcinoma can be caused by:
- Lymphoma.
- Metastases (especially breast).
- Local invasion from pancreatic carcinoma.
- Corrosive ingestion.
- Radiotherapy.
- Crohn's disease.

Case
116

Case 117

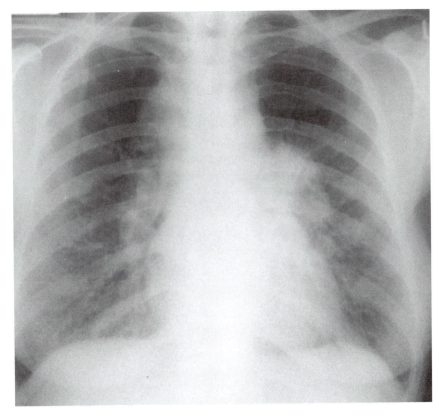

This 25-year-old woman has a history of night sweats and weight loss.

Question

117   What is the likely diagnosis?
- ☐ A   Lymphoma
- ☐ B   Sarcoidosis
- ☐ C   Lung abscess
- ☐ D   Tuberculosis.

Answer overleaf

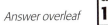

Case 117

Answer

117   A   **Lymphoma**.

Discussion

The chest radiograph shows asymmetrical mediastinal and hilar lymphadenopathy. Subcarinal lymphadenopathy is indicated by loss of visualisation of the azygo-oesophageal line (compare with Case 63, where the line can be clearly seen through the cardiac silhouette). The lungs appear clear.

Intrathoracic lymphadenopathy is the most common manifestation of lymphoma in the thorax and is more common in involvement tends to be bilateral and asymmetrical and most commonly involves anterior mediastinal nodes (refer to Case 63 for a discussion on patterns of mediastinal lymphadenopathy in other conditions). Nodes show a rapid response to radiotherapy and 'eggshell' calcification of lymph nodes may be observed 1–9 years after radiotherapy.

Lung involvement is very unusual without lymphadenopathy.

Case
117

Case
118

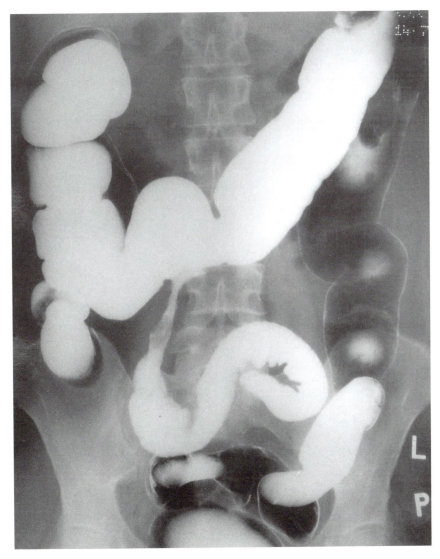

Question

118   What is the likely diagnosis?

☐   A   Crohn's colitis

☐   B   Colonic carcinoma

☐   C   Diverticular disease.

Answer overleaf

Answer

118   A   **Crohn's colitis.**

Discussion

The double contrast barium enema shows an abnormal appearance of the terminal ileum, which is narrowed and irregular, typical of Crohn's disease. Right sacroiliac joint and lumbar spine are normal. There is no evidence of a colonic carcinoma.

Other radiological abnormalities that may be seen in Crohn's disease are strictures which may be single or multiple. Asymmetrical involvement and skip lesions are characteristic.

Disease predominates on the mesenteric border. Ulceration of various degrees (Figure 118A), with the terminal ileum the commonest site. Complications include fistulas, toxic megacolon, carcinoma (less common than in ulcerative colitis), lymphoma, gallstones, sclerosing cholangitis and arthritis.

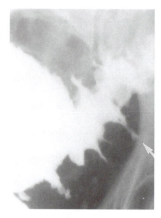

Figure 118A Rose-thorn ulcers (arrow).

Other conditions affecting the terminal ileum are:

- Ulcerative colitis: 10% of those with total colitis have 'backwash' ileitis for up to 25 cm. No ulcers (Figure 118B).
- Tuberculosis (TB): can look identical to Crohn's disease, but predominantly it involves the caecum. Less than 50% have pulmonary TB.
- Lymphoma: may mimic Crohn's disease, but often additional signs are present.
- Less common causes include carcinoid, metastases, ischaemia (rare site) and radiation enteritis.

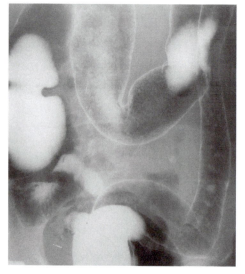

Figure 118B Total colitis in ulcerative colitis leads to a featureless, 'hose-pipe', colon. Rectum involved in 95%.

Case 118

Case 119

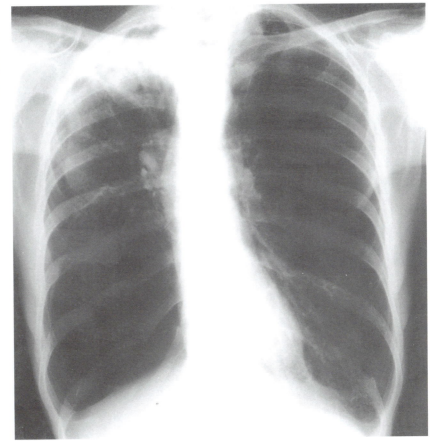

This 50-year-old man has haemoptysis.

Question

119   What is the likely cause?

   ☐ **A** Pancoast's tumour

   ☐ **B** Acute tuberculosis

   ☐ **C** Mycetoma

   ☐ **D** Mesothelioma.

Answer overleaf

Case 119

Answer

119   C   **Mycetoma.**

Discussion

There is a mycetoma (aspergilloma, fungus ball) within a pre-existing cavity in the right upper lobe (at the level of the medial end of the clavicle). Note the rounded mass of soft tissue density lying within the cavity. There is a characteristic air-crescent sign surrounding the fungus ball which does not completely fill the cavity. This sign, although not specific to mycetoma, strongly suggests the diagnosis; another useful diagnostic sign is that a fungus ball moves with patient positioning.

Pleural thickening of up to 2 cm adjacent to the cavity is a frequent finding of *Aspergillus* superinfection and may be the first sign in a patient with a pre-existing lung cavity. CT scanning demonstrates these features even better.

The fungus ball may calcify.

Although the pulmonary cavities are usually due to old, healed pulmonary tuberculosis (note the right upper zone fibrosis, elevation of the right hilum and hilar nodal calcification) other causes include sarcoidosis, ankylosing spondylitis and bronchiectasis. In this patient there are also large emphysematous bullae in the right lower and left upper zones, respectively.

Case 120

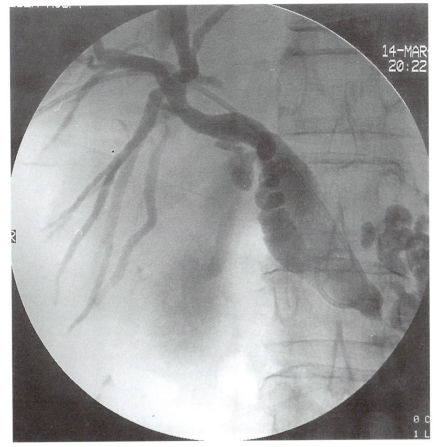

Questions

120a   What type of investigation is this?

☐   A   Hepatic angiogramphy

☐   B   Percutaneous transhepatic cholangiogramphy (PTC)

☐   C   ERCP (Endoscopic Retrograde Cholangia Pancreatography.

120b   What radiological abnormality is shown?

☐   A   Obstruction of the distal common bile duct

☐   B   Obstruction of the intrahepatic ducts

☐   C   Biliary leak

☐   D   Filling defects within the common bile duct.

120c   What is the cause of this appearance?

☐   A   Gallstones

☐   B   Sclerosing cholangitis

☐   C   Chronic pancreatitis.

Answer overleaf   Case 120

Answers

120a B **Percutaneous transhepatic cholagiogram (PTC).**

120b A **Obstruction of the distal common bile duct.**

120c C **Chronic pancreatitis.**

Discussion

The PTC is performed by passing a needle percutaneously into the liver under local anaesthetic. Contrast is injected into the biliary tree. (A catheter can be inserted to drain an obstructed system as shown above.) This PTC demonstrates obstruction of the distal common bile duct with dilatation of the intrahepatic ducts, cystic duct, common hepatic and common bile duct. The level of obstruction is within the pancreas with abrupt tapering of the common bile duct. Multiple densities (i.e. of similar density to the dense contrast material within the bile duct), consistent with calcifications, are seen in the region of the head of pancreas, projected over the left lateral border of the lumbar vertebrae, consistent with chronic calcific pancreatitis. Such calcifications are seen more clearly on the preliminary plain abdominal film before to the injection of contrast.

Causes of distal common bile duct obstruction include:
* Calculi: single or multiple intraluminal filling defects that may change position.
* Malignant tumours: including cholangiocarcinoma, ampullary tumours and carcinoma of the pancreas. Compression by enlarged lymph nodes.
* Chronic pancreatitis: look for pancreatic calcifications.
* Inflammatory benign strictures, e.g. due to recurrent pyogenic cholangitis, pancreatic pseudocyst, etc.

Case 121

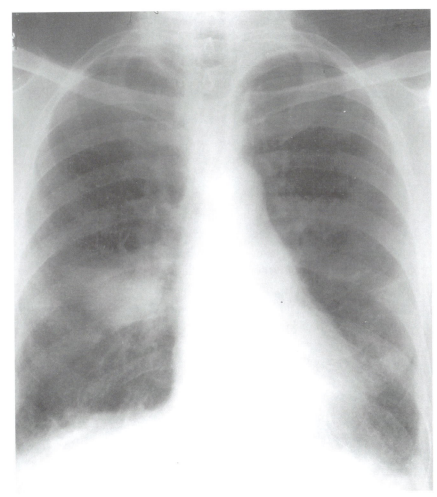

Chest X-ray of a patient with bronchogenic carcinoma.

Question

121   What is the likely association?

☐ A Previous radiotherapy

☐ B Alpha-1 antitrypsin deficiency

☐ C Asbestos exposure.

Answer overleaf

Case 121

Answer

121   C   **Asbestos exposure.**

Discussion

The chest X-ray demonstrates pleural thickening and calcified pleural plaque (right hemidiaphragm). There is a fine reticular pattern in both lower zones. A large irregular non-cavitating pulmonary mass is projected over the inferior pole of the right hilum.

The X-ray features are of asbestosis and bronchogenic carcinoma.

Plaques occur on the parietal pleura and are seen in 50% of patients exposed to asbestos (not before 20 years or more have elapsed). They tend to be multiple and favour the lower hemithorax. The interstitial, reticular pattern compatible with fibrosis (asbestosis) is typically basal. There is an increased incidence of bronchogenic carcinoma in smokers with asbestosis.

Other findings include mesothelioma (80% of all mesotheliomas are associated with asbestosis) and pleural effusions.

Pleural calcification may also be due to an old empyema, haemothorax (typically unilateral) or talc exposure (similar appearance to asbestos exposure).

Case **122**

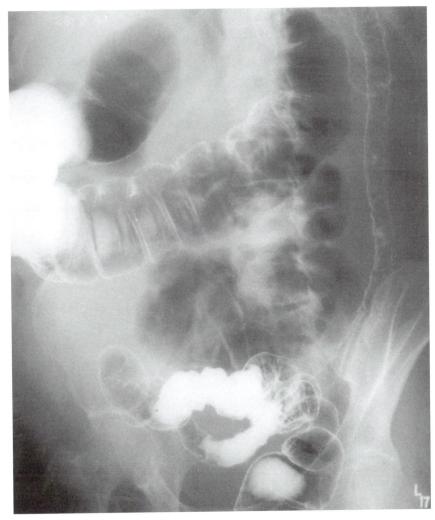

This 72-year-old patient has acute abdominal pain and rectal bleeding.

Question

122   What is the likely cause?

☐ A   Crohn's disease
☐ B   Ulcerative colitis
☐ C   Ischaemic colitis
☐ D   Diverticulitis
☐ E   Carcinoma of the colon.

Answer overleaf   Case **122**

Answer

122   C   **Ischaemic colitis**.

Discussion

The double contrast barium enema shows a continuous long narrowed segment extending from the splenic flexure to the sigmoid colon with fine mucosal ulceration. There is no evidence of associated malignancy or diverticular disease.

The radiological findings in conjunction with the clinical history make ischaemic colitis the most likely diagnosis.

The descending colon (90%) and splenic flexure (80%) are the commonest sites of involvement in ischaemic colitis.

Plain film changes include thumb printing (marginal indentations on the mesenteric side), lack of haustration and narrowing. Barium enema is the definitive investigation (abnormal in 90% of patients) and features include superficial ulcerations, thumb printing (due to submucosal haemorrhage and oedema), and rigidity.

Poor prognostic features are toxic megacolon (colonic calibre greater than 5.5 cm), pneumoperitoneum and gas in the portal vein. Intramural gas may be seen and is linear in configuration rather than spherical as in pneumatosis coli (Figure 49A).

Causes of toxic megacolon are:
• Inflammatory: ulcerative colitis, Crohn's disease and pseudomembranous colitis.
• Ischaemic colitis.
• Dysentery: amoebiasis, Salmonella.

Case
122

Case 123

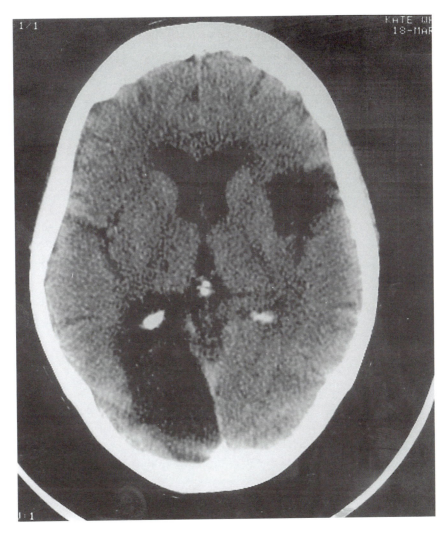

Enhanced CT head scan of a 70-year-old man.

Question

123   What is the diagnosis? Choose *two* answers.
- ☐ A   Left occipital lobe infarct
- ☐ B   Right occipital lobe infarct
- ☐ C   Left frontal lobe infarct
- ☐ D   Right frontal lobe infarct
- ☐ E   Intraventricular haemorrhage.

Answer overleaf

Answer

123   C, D   **Left frontal lobe infarct and right occipital lobe infarct.**

Discussion

There is a well-defined, focal area of decreased attenuation in the left frontoparietal region. There is no associated mass effect and appearances are in keeping with an old infarct (ischaemic lesion) in the left middle cerebral artery territory (the most common territory involved). In addition, there is asymmetrical enlargement of the posterior horn of the right lateral ventricle which is due to a previous right occipital infarct.

The CT appearances of cerebral infarction are time dependent. Unless the infarction is accompanied by haemorrhage in the first 24 hours, CT will detect only 50% of infarcts. Findings include slight hypodensity, minimal mass effect and loss of distinction between grey and white matter.

Mass effect due to oedema is maximal at 3–5 days and gyriform contrast enhancement (when given) is maximal at 2–4 weeks.

Haemorrhage may occur after a few days to 2 weeks due to rebleeding from reperfused, damaged capillaries.

In the chronic stage (by 2–3 months after the event), a well-defined low attenuation area (the same density as CSF) is seen, associated with volume loss (dilatation of adjacent ventricles and sulci).

The high density in the third ventricle and posterior horns of the lateral ventricles are due to calcification of the choroid plexus (not haemorrhage).

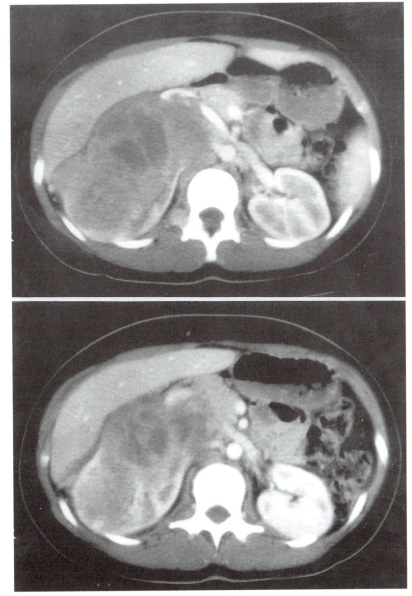

Contrast-enhanced CT scan of the abdomen of a 7-year-old child.

Question

124   What is the most likely diagnosis?

☐   A   Nephroblastoma

☐   B   Neuroblastoma

☐   C   Lymphoma

☐   D   Liver abscess.

Answer overleaf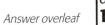

Answer

124   A   **Nephroblastoma** (Wilms' tumour).

Discussion

There is a large soft tissue mass of mixed attenuation arising from the right kidney. It contains low attenuation areas compatible with haemorrhage/necrosis. It extends towards the midline and displaces the right renal artery anteriorly. No calcification is seen. Although not clearly shown on these sections, the right renal vein and IVC were invaded by tumour. Normal liver and left kidney.

This is the commonest abdominal malignancy of childhood with 90% occurring before 8 years of age. They are bilateral in 5% of cases and typically large (average size 12 cm). Calcification is uncommon (5–10%). Five per cent have tumour thrombus in the IVC or right atrium. Ninety per cent have favourable histology.

Plain films may show a bulging flank (75%), loss of the renal outline (66%), enlargement of the renal outline, displacement of bowel gas (50%), loss of psoas outline and calcification.

On IVU (Figure 124A) there is usually calyceal distortion, but in 10% of cases the kidney is not visualised.

Renal cell carcinoma (90% of adult malignant renal tumours) is rare in childhood and carries a worse prognosis than Wilms' tumour.

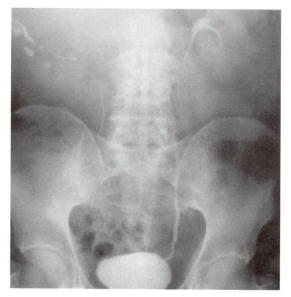

Figure 124A IVU. Right renal cell carcinoma (adult patient) showing calyceal distortion due to an upper pole mass.

Case
124

Case
125

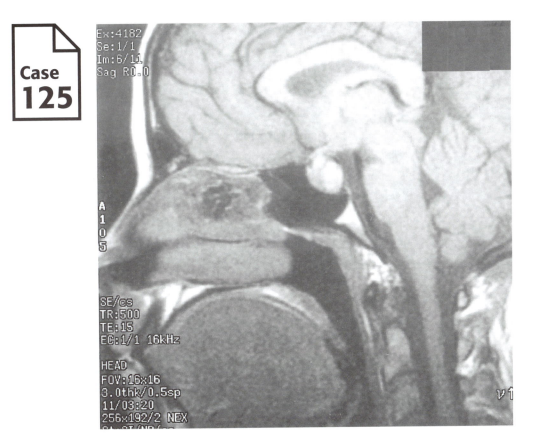

MRI scan of a 25-year-old woman.

Question

125   What abnormality is shown?

☐ A   Pituitary macroadenoma

☐ B   Pituitary microadenoma

☐ C   Empty sella syndrome.

Answer overleaf

Case
125

Answer

125 A **Pituitary macroadenoma.**

Discussion

This T1-weighted sagittal MRI brain scan without contrast shows enlargement of the pituitary fossa by a large pituitary mass, with suprasellar extension up to the optic chiasm.

MRI, with its multiplanar capability, is the optimal imaging technique for this region. On T1-weighted images, pituitary tumours tend to be of slightly lower signal intensity than the adjacent anterior pituitary tissue, a difference that is emphasised after intravenous contrast enhancement, i.e. the adenoma does not enhance, but normal adjacent pituitary gland enhances substantially. The size of tumour at presentation varies from a few millimetres with adrenocorticotrophic hormone-producing adenomas to very large, in the case of non-functioning tumours or those that produce prolactin (as in this case) or growth hormone. A macroadenoma is defined as a tumour of diameter greater than 1 cm. There are no imaging features to distinguish between different types of adenoma.

Large tumours may extend upwards into the suprasellar cistern and compress the optic chiasm and hypothalamus. Invasive tumours grow into the cavernous sinus and may invade adjacent brain substance.

Case
125

Case
126

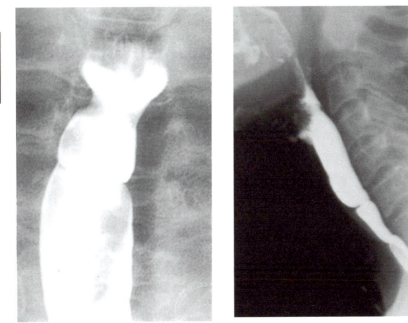

This 45-year-old woman presents with dysphagia.

Question

126　What does the barium swallow show?

   □ A Carcinoma of the oesophagus

   □ B Oesophageal web

   □ C Oesophageal ulceration.

Answer overleaf

Case
126

Answer

126   B   **Oesophageal web**: a smooth thin lucent band (occasionally multiple) arising from the anterior wall of the upper oesophagus just below the cricopharyngeal impression. It is seen opposite C5/C6 on the lateral view.

Discussion

Oesophageal webs are semicircular membranes of variable size and are usually an incidental finding of no clinical importance, typically in the upper oesophagus. They are common in patients with dysphagia owing to concomitant functional abnormalities of swallowing, but may themselves be a cause for dysphagia when large enough to produce obstruction.

Post-cricoid webs are associated with the Plummer–Vinson syndrome. The relationship to carcinoma is controversial.

Webs may occur as a complication of certain skin diseases, including epidermolysis bullosa and pemphigoid.

Index